INSIDE OURSELVES

INSIDE OURSELVES

HOW OUR BODIES WORK

CHRISTOPHER BELL

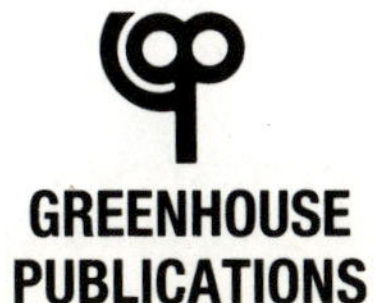

GREENHOUSE
PUBLICATIONS

First published in 1989 by
Greenhouse Publications Pty Ltd
122–126 Ormond Road
Elwood Victoria 3184 Australia

Designed by Sandra Nobes
Typeset in Australia by Solo Typesetting
in 11/13 pt Garamond condensed
Printed in Hong Kong

National Library of Australia
Cataloguing-in-publication data:

Bell, Christopher, 1941–
Inside ourselves, how our body works.

Includes index.
ISBN 0 86436 214 5.

1. Body, Human. 2. Anatomy, Human. I. Title.

612

COVER INSERT: *Life-size human model made in Germany around 1900.*

COVER BACKGROUND: *Nerve cells identified by use of an immunological label are coded by computer. Different colours denote different intensities of label.*

Table of Contents

	Preface	vii
1	*From Galen to Gene Cloning*	1
2	*The Keys to Action*	15
3	*Blood is Richer than Water*	24
4	*Staying in Circulation*	33
5	*A Breath of Fresh Air*	44
6	*Stoking Up the Furnace*	57
7	*The Quintessential Filter*	67
8	*Keeping a Cool Head*	77
9	*The New and the Old*	86
10	*Looking Outwards . . .*	95
11	*. . . and Looking Inwards*	105
	Sources of Illustrations	114
	Index	117

'A modern poet has characterised the personality of Art and the impersonality of Science as follows: Art is I; Science is We.'

Claude Bernard

Preface

All over the world medical scientists are involved in studying physiology, that is the way in which our bodies work. Through the centuries, physiological knowledge has advanced at an uneven and unpredictable pace, usually in tiny stages, but sometimes in quantum leaps. Breakthroughs in other related disciplines like chemistry and physics have often provided sudden insights into, for example, enzyme actions and electrical impulses in nerves. New technologies like microscopes and X-rays periodically provide new ways of looking at the body. But just as many advances can be attributed to unusual insight or to sheer good luck.

This book has been written with two aims, which might at first sight seem contradictory. The first is to help readers with no background in biology realise that our bodies function in quite logical ways, and that most common illnesses can be understood by appreciating that they are due to a malfunction of one or other of our organ systems.

The second aim is to dispel the myth that we already know virtually everything about how the human body works. In fact, despite the enormous amount of information that has been collected over the years, we even now know very little about some aspects of physiological control. Continued basic research offers the only way in which, eventually, we may be able to prevent most human diseases, rather than just treating them. As it becomes increasingly difficult to provide adequate hospital care even in advanced Western communities, the relatively small amount of funding used in basic research becomes more and more attractive as an investment in the future of humanity.

The series of articles on which this book is based was conceived in 1985 following discussions with Sally White, who was then Science Editor of the *Age* newspaper. I am indebted to her for encouragement and for her help in making my pedantic scientific writing more journalistically acceptable. My wife Christine also helped to refine the text, and acted as adviser with the numerous illustrations that come from the unique collection held by the State Library of Victoria.

Cam Knuckey provided the original drawings that appear on pages 21, 70 and 107, and Reinier Mann photographed many of the laboratory specimens. For their help in obtaining other illustrations, I am grateful to Professor Harold Attwood, the curator of the Medical History Museum, and Dr Daine Alcorn, of the Department of Anatomy, both in the University of Melbourne. Karen Cosgriff and Cathy Smith also gave invaluable assistance in final preparation of the book. As well, various colleagues and readers have helped by pointing out errors, ambiguities and misprints in the original newspaper articles: any that remain are my fault, not theirs.

Christopher Bell
Melbourne, April, 1988

Chapter One

From Galen to Gene Cloning

The cell is the basic building block of a complex animal like man. Each of us starts off as a single cell, the fertilised egg, and this divides repeatedly into two, four, eight and so on. As the number of cells grows, particular groups of them become specialised for particular functions, a process called differentiation. Some cells become muscle, specialised to produce movement; others become nerve, which conducts electricity, or epithelium, for controlling the movement of various molecules between different body compartments, or connective tissue, to hold all the other cells together.

When a lot of cells of the same type are grouped together, they are called a tissue. In turn, some or all of the four tissue types join together to make up the functional units of the body, the organs, such as brain, lung and heart. Finally, several organs with related functions can be regarded as forming organ systems. For instance, the heart and the blood vessels joined to it make up the cardiovascular system.

The body is made up of many millions of cells, within which a variety of chemical reactions, collectively called metabolism, occur. Metabolic processes depend on the continual movement of foodstuffs and oxygen into the cells, and the continual removal of waste products. These movements rely in turn on the diffusion of molecules from areas where they are highly concentrated to areas where they are more dilute.

Diffusion is a rapid process only over very short distances, so there is a practical limit to how large a cell can grow. An elephant is far bigger than a mouse, and contains many more cells, but each mouse cell is about the same size as the same sort of cell in an elephant. Most cells in our bodies have diameters of about one to two hundredths of a millimetre: that is, up to ten of them would fit in the thickness of a page of this book.

Cells carry out two sorts of activity. The first of these is the series of basic metabolic processes that are necessary for the cell itself to live, and which are quite similar for all types of cell. The second activity is the performance of the particular function for which the cell is specialised, such as the production of movement by muscle cells. In this way, the body is like a society, with all individuals carrying out their everyday routines like sleeping and eating, but also having specific jobs that serve the community's needs. The type of job on which a particular cell is employed determines both its appearance and its chemistry. So, for example, red blood cells have a flat, disk shape, which provides the maximum surface area for exchange of oxygen, as well as containing the haemoglobin protein essential for carrying oxygen.

Many of the specialised activities of cells have the role of contributing to the maintenance of a constant fluid environment in which all the cells live, the extracellular fluid. For instance, contraction of muscle cells of the heart maintains the flow of oxygen-bearing blood around the body, while contraction of the chest muscles opens and shuts the lungs and maintains the exchange of oxygen between the air and the bloodstream. Both systems are therefore helping to keep a constant oxygen concentration in the extracellular fluid. But, in order for these regulating functions to be effective, the cells have to be told continually about the amount of oxygen that is present. The physiological stability of the body therefore depends on internal signalling systems, such as nerves and hormones, as well as on systems that respond to these signals.

The first comprehensive view of physiology was put forward by Galen, a Greek physician to the Roman emperor Marcus Aurelius in the second century AD. To Galen, the world was made up of four elements: fire, air, earth and water; four corresponding constituents of the body, called humours, provided the full variety of human personalities. Blood (thought to come from the liver) gave a happy, or sanguine, character, black bile (from the spleen) a melancholic one; yellow bile from the gall bladder made one irritable and phlegm from the lungs produced apathy. All one had to do to explain anyone's personality problems was to suggest an imbalance between these influences.

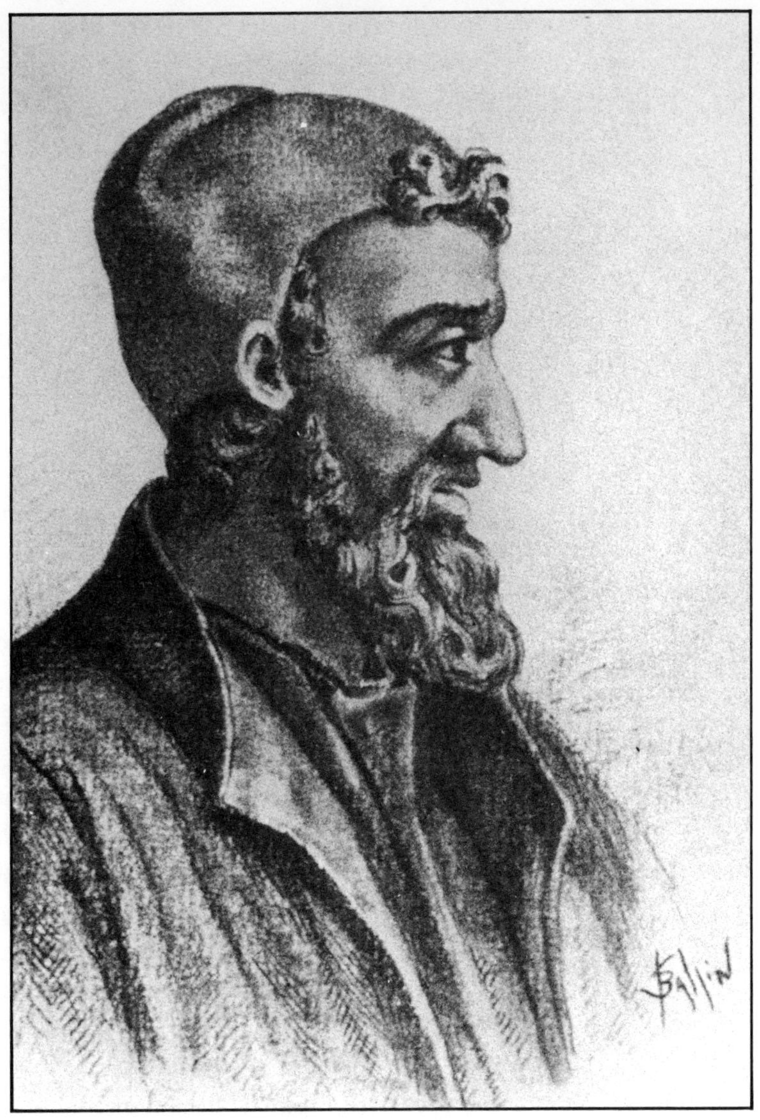

The Greek physician, Galen, was the first to propose a coherent system of human physiology.

Modern psychiatrists probably regret that their task is not so straightforward.

Rather than the blood being pumped around the body from arteries to veins, Galen believed that it ebbed and flowed between the liver and the veins, through which it carried 'natural spirits' to nourish the various tissues. A much smaller amount of blood travelled to the heart, where it penetrated through pores between right and left ventricles, and mixed with air from the lungs to become a gas called 'vital spirits'. This was pumped through the pulsating arteries to provide heat to the body.

Some blood also travelled to the brain, where it was changed into 'animal spirits'. This flowed out to all parts of the body through hollow nerves. Contraction of the muscles was due to an inflow of 'animal spirits', inflating them like a balloon being blown up. (It is worth noting that the word 'animal' here is derived from the Latin word for the soul, *animus*, and does not actually refer to animals.)

Galen based some of his ideas on those of earlier Greek philosophers, and some on his observations of dissected dead animals. But, without experimental evidence as well, these observations were more misleading than helpful. For instance, we know that after death blood drains from the arteries into the veins. But when Galen saw that the arteries of dead animals were empty, he interpreted this as evidence that the arteries carry gas rather than blood.

Nevertheless, Galen's teachings were accepted as absolute truth for nearly 1500 years. There were two reasons for this. For one thing, however unlikely Galen's ideas seem in retrospect, the real answers to questions like how a nerve works could never be obtained until technological advances in chemistry and physics allowed the necessary experiments to be carried out. The second factor was that in Western societies neither human dissection nor animal experiments were widely accepted until the sixteenth century. So it was difficult to acquire information on either the structure or the behaviour of living bodies.

Even when this information became available, Galen's ideas attracted such respect that people were reluctant to contradict them. In about 1500 Leonardo da Vinci drew very accurate pictures of the heart, in which he showed the absence of the intraventricular pores that would be necessary for movement of 'vital spirits', and the presence of the heart valves that suggest one-way movement of blood into the heart from the veins and out into the arteries. However, his preconceptions were so strong that he managed to ignore the conclusion which is obvious to us today. At about the same time, the anatomist Vesalius also noticed the absence of pores in the heart. He drew the correct conclusions, but when he tried to publicise them he was forced to resign from his university post.

However, in the early seventeenth century, a report contradicting Galen appeared which was so convincing that it could not be ignored. William Harvey, a young Englishman who had studied medicine in Padua, returned to a lectureship at the Royal College of Physicians and began to lecture on the bloodstream in the year that Shakespeare died. Twelve years later he published a

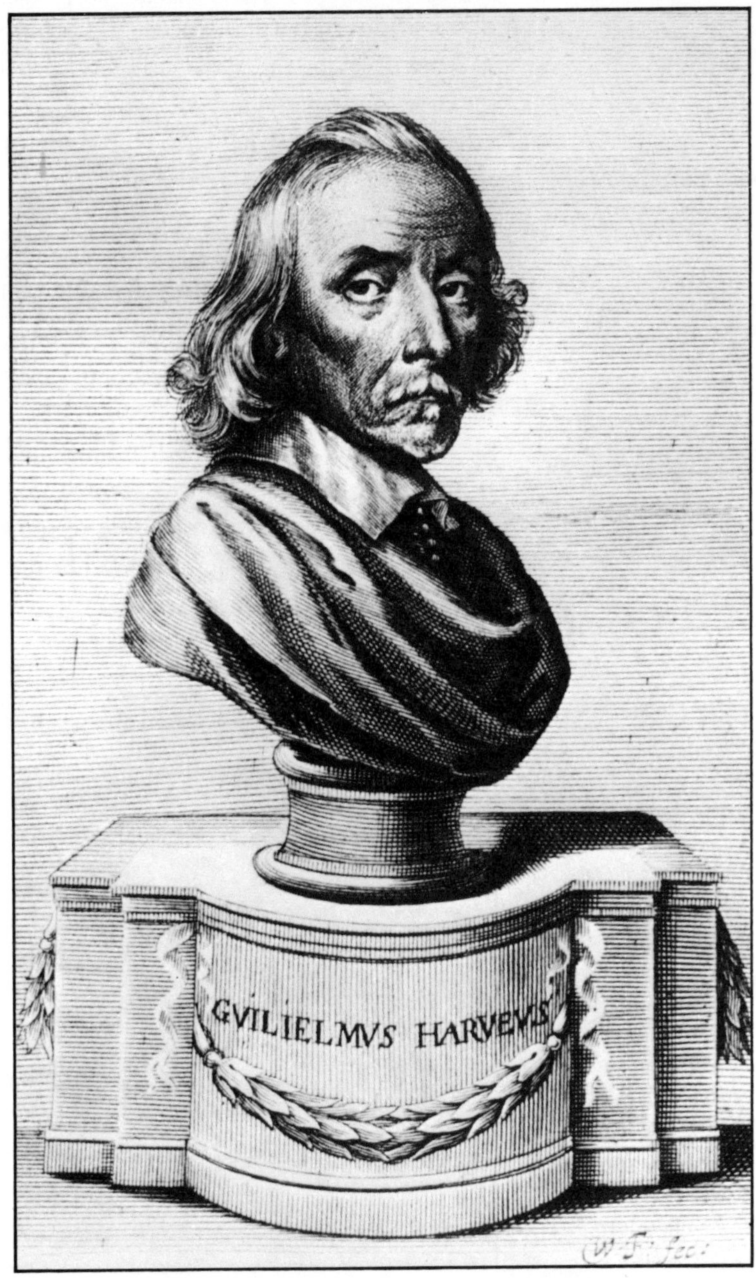

William Harvey revolutionised medical science by proving that blood circulated around the body.

book of just seventy-two pages, *On the Circulation of the Blood.* Not only did this refute a view that had been dogma for over a thousand years, but it was the earliest example of the quantitative approach to research which has been the pivot of scientific endeavour ever since.

Before Harvey, scientists had only ever made straightforward observations of naturally occurring processes. Harvey, however, had learnt from the astronomer Galileo in Italy the power of quantitative and deductive reasoning. Now, he looked at the effects of manipulating natural processes, made precise measurements of the effects and then reasoned out the most likely explanation.

First, he drained the blood from a dead sheep to determine the total blood volume. Next, he measured how much blood was moved out of the heart with a single beat, and showed that the amount that would be moved in an hour was much more than the total blood volume. The blood must therefore recirculate.

By opening the chests of cold-blooded animals like frogs, in which the rate of heart beat is much slower than in mammals, Harvey could see that the pulsing of the arteries was caused by the heart beating, rather than being produced by the vessels themselves. He could also see that the arteries carried blood and

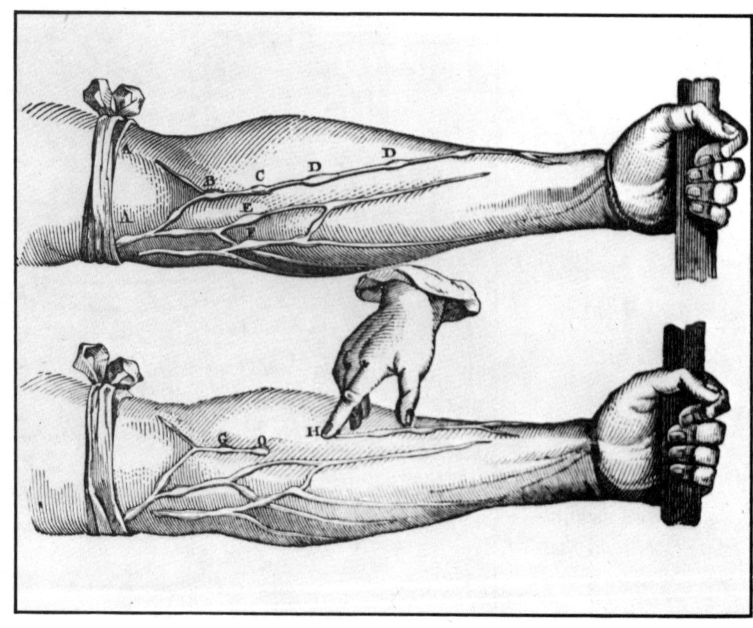

One of the vital pieces of evidence in Harvey's proof of blood circulation was the fact that blood in the veins of the arm flows only in one direction, towards the heart; valves stop it travelling back towards the hand, as demonstrated here in one of the illustrations from Harvey's book.

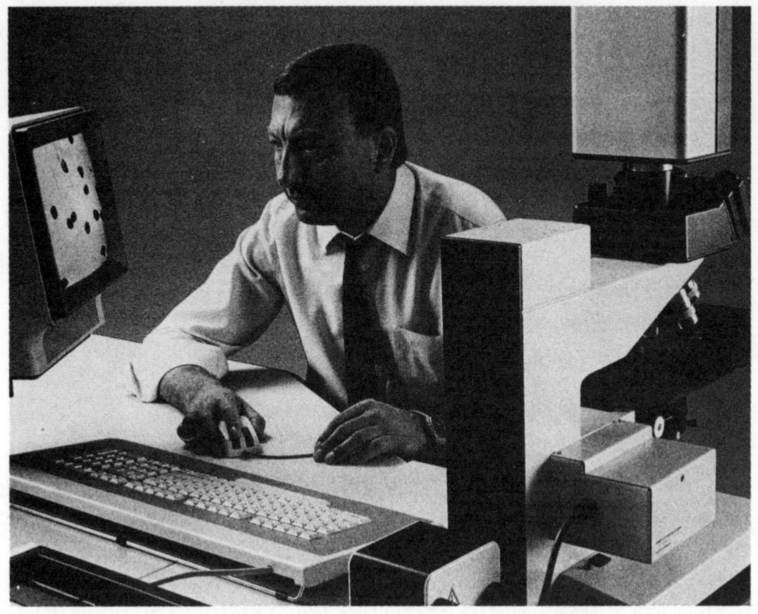

The modern research microscope is often linked to a video camera and a computer, allowing sophisticated analysis of cell properties.

not gas. Finally, he demonstrated that in the human arm the veins contained one-way valves, so that blood could move along them only towards the heart, not away from it as required by Galen's teachings. The heart was obviously responsible for forcing blood around the body, from arteries to veins.

There was one thing that Harvey could not determine by experiment: the way in which the blood passed from arteries to veins. The explanation for this had to wait forty years, for the invention of the microscope. Then the Italian, Malpighi, and the Dutchman, Leeuwenhoek, actually saw blood cells moving through the tiny capillaries that link the arterial and the venous systems. The circuit was complete.

Harvey's experiments dismissed to a great extent the Galenic ideas of 'natural spirits' and 'vital spirits', but they did not touch on 'animal spirits' and the function of the nerves. One of the first men to experiment in this area was Giovanni Borelli, professor of mathematics at Pisa, who in the 1650s slit a contracted muscle under water and saw that no gas escaped. Unfortunately, he only concluded from this that the 'animal spirit' causing muscle expansion was liquid rather than gaseous. Then in about 1670 the Dutchman, Swammerdam, sealed a frog's muscle into a chamber which was connected to a glass tube containing a drop of water. He saw that when the muscle contracted, the water drop did not move. Therefore, although the muscle appeared to swell when it contracted, it could not have actually increased in volume.

Swammerdam persuaded Leeuwenhoek to use his microscope to see if cross sections of nerves contained the canals needed for the flow of 'animal spirits'. At first he reported that no canals existed, but the Galenists insisted that he look more carefully. Leeuwenhoek knew nothing about preparing animal tissues for microscopy – neither would anybody else for another hundred years – so, when he looked at his crudely prepared nerves for long enough, he saw the interior of each nerve dry out, leaving what did appear to be a canal. Galen seemed to be vindicated! Swammerdam was a disappointed man, and perhaps Leeuwenhoek's failure made him mistrust his own judgement. In any case, the results of his crucial experiment with the frog muscle were not published until seventy years later, long after his death.

A nerve trunk cut in cross-section shows the outlines of the individual nerve fibres. Here a special dye has been used to show up the cytoplasm inside each fibre. Failure to see this led the seventeenth century microscopist, Leeuwenhoek, to conclude that nerves were empty tubes.

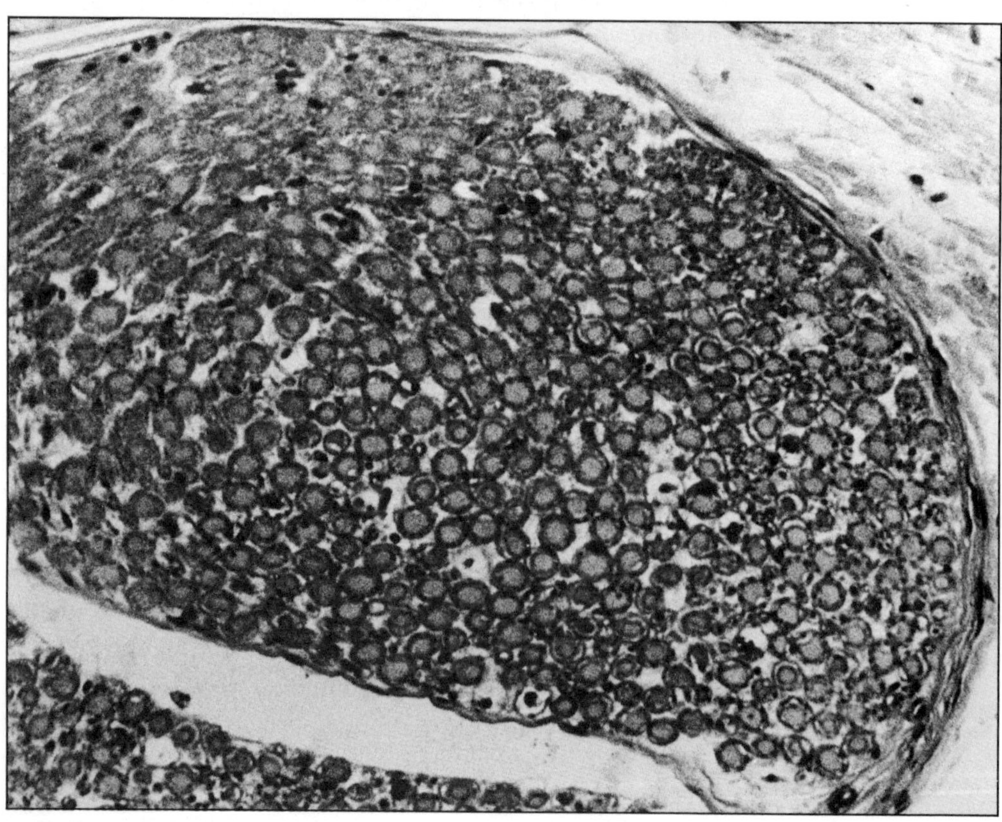

After Harvey, more than a century passed before the next great advance in knowledge of the circulation took place. In 1732 an amateur botanist called Stephen Hales was measuring sap pressure in plants by means of vertical tubes inserted into the stems. He reasoned that a similar approach could be used to determine blood pressures in animals. Hales inserted a long vertical pipe into an artery of a horse. He saw that blood rose in the pipe to a height of about eight feet, balancing the pressure within the artery. An eight-foot column of blood is about equal to a 180 millimetre column of mercury: in other words, the horse's blood pressure was about 180 millimetres of mercury. Hales also saw that the pressure rose and fell with the heart beat and with breathing, and that the pressure in veins was very much lower than in arteries. What he could not do was to confirm his findings in man. This had to wait another 150 years for the invention of the arm cuff and the mercury manometer, still used by doctors today.

Within a few years of Hales's experiments, the scientific renaissance of the eighteenth century was in full flight, and the phenomenon of electricity was becoming well documented. Men like Galvani and Volta were making devices with which electric shocks could be applied to living tissues. At last it became possible to study the concept of animal spirits in earnest.

This final era of research began with the French physiologist, Claude Bernard. Bernard found that electrical impulses applied to the nerves that accompanied a blood vessel caused it to contract, reducing blood flow. Cutting the same nerve caused blood vessel relaxation and an increased blood flow. Thus the normal resistance of vessels to flow through them must be adjusted by the activity of the nerves.

Bernard was also intrigued by the South American arrow poison, curare, which was known to paralyse animals and people. He found that the muscle contraction produced by electrical stimulation of a nerve was prevented by curare. After poisoning, shocks applied to the muscle were also unable to cause contraction. Bernard concluded from this observation that communication between nerve and muscle was not due to electricity, but to some other sort of process. In fact, there was no contraction because Bernard's source of electricity was too weak to

The nineteenth century physiologist and playwright, Claude Bernard, is often regarded as the founder of modern physiology. As well as making many crucial discoveries about how the nervous system controls the body, he was the first to realise that the main role of most of our bodily functions is to maintain a stable environment in which our cells can survive.

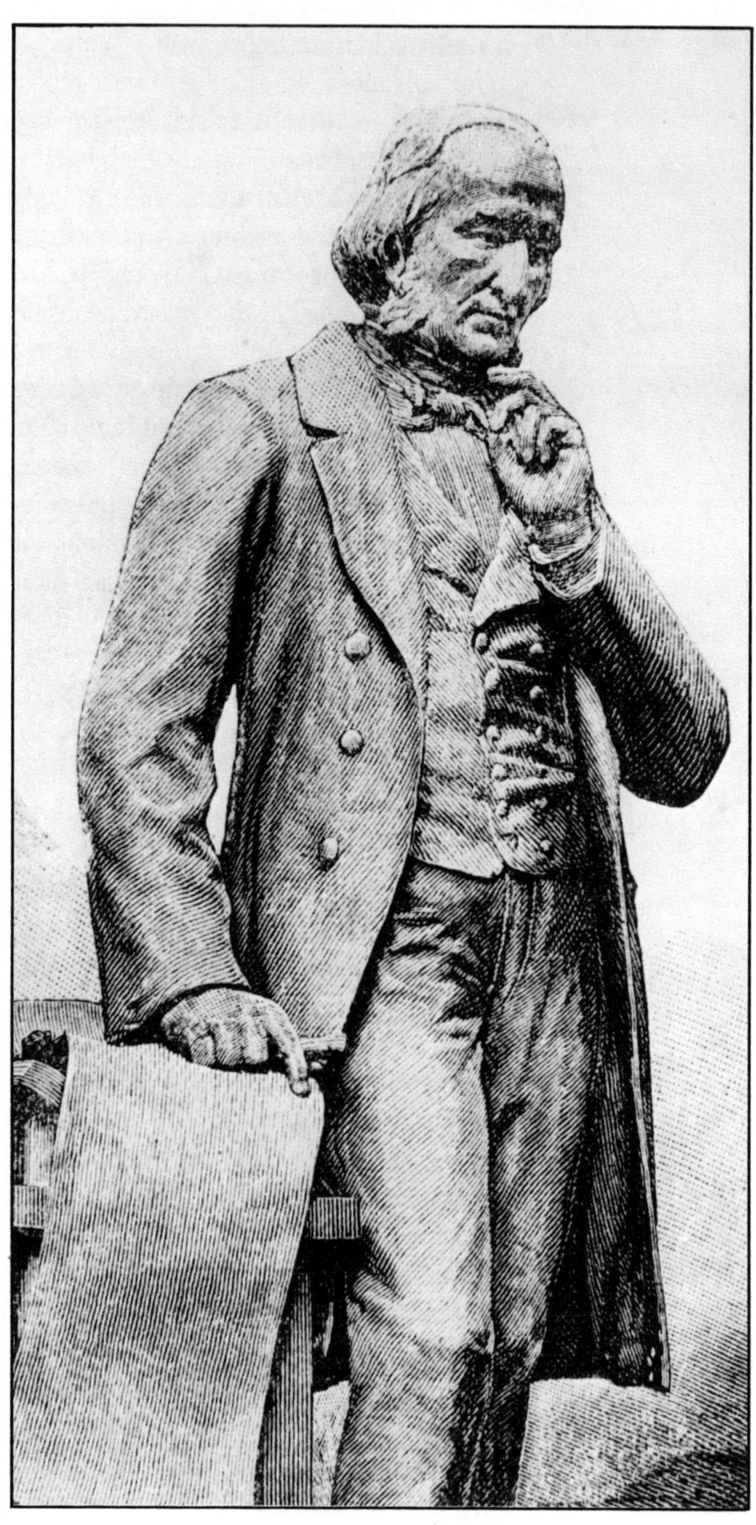

excite the muscle cells. Nevertheless, his suggestion sowed in the minds of scientists the seed of an idea that nerve and muscle might be separate entities which communicated by some specialised means.

The basis of this means of communication makes up the last part of our story. In 1905 a Cambridge medical student named Thomas Renton Elliott observed that muscles contracted in the presence of certain chemicals from the body, even after the nerves had been removed. He suggested that the nerves might normally release a similar chemical onto the muscle. Other scientists soon noticed further situations in which the responses of various types of muscle to nerve impulses were mimicked by applying particular biological substances.

The proof of Elliott's idea came from Otto Loewi in 1921. In a brilliantly simple experiment, Loewi collected fluid from around a frog's heart after electrically stimulating the vagus nerve, which causes the heart to slow its rate of beating. When Loewi applied some of the bathing fluid to a second heart, its beat also weakened. The release from nerves of a chemical that affected muscle had been proven at last, and the final bastion of Galenic science fell.

Since the time of the experiments I have described, an enormous amount of information has accumulated concerning the blood circulation and the control of muscle activity, as well as other areas of physiology. Most of this new information has been made possible by new developments in technology, allowing measurements to be made far more accurately, and providing techniques for assessing previously unmeasurable parameters.

One example of this progress is the recent development of gene cloning as an experimental tool. It is difficult to investigate the actions of many hormones and neurotransmitters, because they are present only in minute quantities – in some cases only fractions of a one-millionth of a gram of the whole body. However, the molecular biologist is now able to sift the genetic material in selected types of cell, and remove the section that controls production of a particular molecule: for instance, a hormone. This genetic information is then grafted into a virus, which multiplies rapidly and produces large amounts of the hormone for experimental study.

Gene cloning also offers new hope for understanding the biochemical basis of poorly understood hereditary illnesses like Huntington's disease. If the gene that carries the disease can be isolated and cloned, then it will be possible to identify the substance whose production it controls.

The advances of modern medical biology allow us to say with confidence that personality is not governed by Galen's four humours, at least in the simple way that he thought. Years of documenting the behaviour of patients with known areas of brain damage has taught us much about the pathways that contribute to the expression of certain personality characteristics. We have many drugs by which mood and behaviour can be altered in predictable ways. Nonetheless, we still do not seem to be much closer than Galen to understanding those properties of the human brain which provide our individual personalities, or our capacities for thought and artistic expression.

Even with topics that are generally thought to be fully understood, there are sometimes surprising new discoveries. One example concerns the capacity of the adult brain to grow. It has been accepted for many years that birds and mammals are born with all the brain cells they will ever have. Tasks like memory and learning have all been thought to be carried out using the same set of cells present when we are babies. Yet in 1984 biologists found that in canaries the numbers of brain cells related to song production increase by tens of thousands at the beginning of each mating season, and that at the end of the mating season all these cells die again.

The importance of this finding is enormous. It indicates that there is some trigger signal that stimulates the growth of new brain cells in an adult vertebrate. If an equivalent signal can be identified for the human brain, this might at last provide a way to alter injury or stroke damage.

New discoveries of a similarly revolutionary nature continue to be made in all areas of physiology, and continue to challenge our accepted beliefs about the body. They illustrate why physiology remains a cornerstone of medical research, and why physiologists can approach their task with continued enthusiasm and wonderment.

THE ACCELERATING DEVELOPMENT OF PHYSIOLOGICAL KNOWLEDGE ABOUT THE NERVOUS SYSTEM

200 AD	*Galen evokes animal spirits as basis for neural system function*
1670	*Swammerdam proves that muscle does not swell when it contracts*
1780	*Galvani shows that electrical impulses activate nerves*
1850	*Bernard uses curare to block nerve-muscle communication*
1890	*Ramon y Cajal uses microscopic studies to propose that the nervous system consists of separate nerve cells*
1905	**Elliott proposes the existence of chemical neurotransmission between these cells**
1921	*Loewi confirms it*
1930s	**Existence of two separate chemical neurotransmitters confirmed**
1940s	*Selective drug molecules are synthesised for manipulating neurotransmission*
	Number of known chemical neurotransmitters extended to three
1950s	*Development of the electronmicroscope and electronic techniques allow the details of neurotransmission to be measured*
	Three more neurotransmitters suggested to exist in brain
1960s	*Development of more selective drug molecules allows the biochemical details of neurotransmission to be studied*
	New microscopic techniques allow nerves containing specific neurotransmitters to be traced
1970s	*Introduction of immunological tools for studying nerve cell biochemistry*

►

	Discovery of biologically active peptide molecules in nerves
	Interactions of nerve cells studied in tissue culture
1980s	*Gene cloning allows biological molecules to be synthesised for experimental and therapeutic use*
	Development of CAT and PET scans allows non-invasive brain studies
	List of possible neurotransmitters in brain reaches 50

Chapter Two

The Keys to Action

Take an eye-dropper filled with ink and squeeze one drop into a large glass of water. Instantly, the drop loses its outline and grows larger. But only after a much longer time will it have spread evenly throughout the water. This tells us that diffusion is a very fast process over short distances, and a very slow one when the distance involved is long. Although communication between the different parts of a tiny animal like an amoeba can rely on diffusion, it could not be a suitable mechanism for communication between the parts of a large animal like man. Instead, large animals have developed specialised internal communication systems. Two of these, the blood circulation and the lungs, serve to transport nutrients and wastestuffs around the body. The third, the nerves, serves to transport information.

When you or I pick up a hot object by mistake, we know about it very quickly, and can let it go again within a fraction of a second. To be useful, therefore, nerves must carry information rapidly, and electrical impulses are the only mechanism by which this rapidity can be achieved.

Electricity travelling along power lines is created by the movement of negatively charged electrons within the metal. Electricity in nerves, by contrast, is created by the movement of positively charged atoms called ions, which diffuse between the inside and the outside of the nerve cell through tiny holes in the cell surface membrane and change the voltage difference across it. Most of the electrical current that is produced in a nerve is carried by ions of sodium and potassium.

Nerves have been likened to submarine cables, and this analogy has some truth in it. Both are submerged in a fluid that is electrically conductive, and both carry electrical currents that are protected from the surrounding fluid by a layer of insulation.

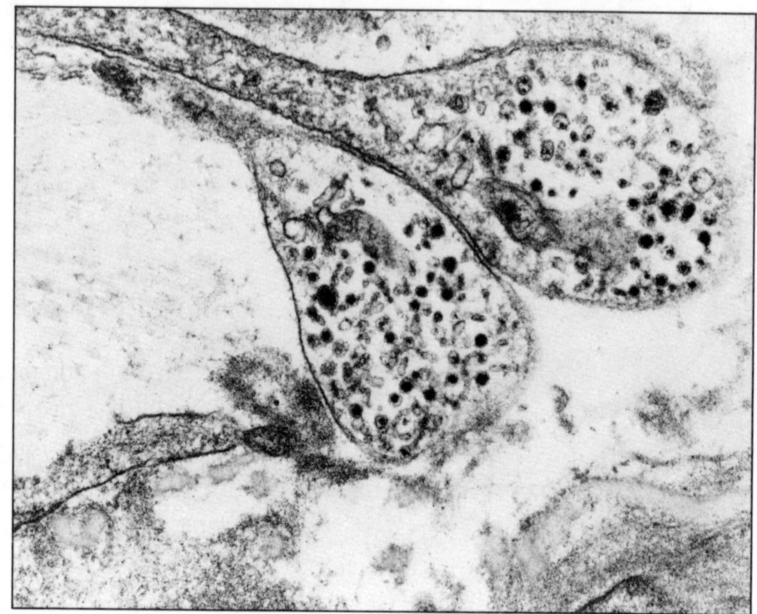

In the electron microscope, two nerve axons are seen to approach the muscle cells of a blood vessel which lies in the lower right hand corner of the picture. The numerous small round objects in the axons are vesicles filled with neuro-transmitter, which is stained black. It will be released onto the blood vessel when the nerves are excited by an action potential.

Here, however, the similarity ends. The metal filaments that make up a cable conduct electricity very easily (that is, they have a very low resistance to current flow), and the insulating plastic around the cable is so efficient that none of the current leaks out. The cable can therefore convey electrical information for thousands of kilometres.

Nerves, on the other hand, must be slightly leaky, because the production of an electric current requires movement of ions between inside and outside. For this reason, a current does not travel evenly along the nerve but progressively leaks out into the surrounding fluid. As cables, then, nerves are very inefficient. So they need some special mechanism to overcome this inefficiency. The mechanism is known as the action potential, or 'spike'.

Imagine what happens if you hold a lighted match under a sheet of paper. When the part of the paper just over the match becomes hot enough, it catches fire, and the fire spreads as it warms up the surrounding paper. A rather similar sequence of events occurs during the action potential, but here electrical rather than temperature changes are involved. When the voltage difference between the inside and the outside of a nerve cell is lowered, holes that are just slightly larger than a sodium ion open in the cell membrane, and sodium rushes into the nerve.

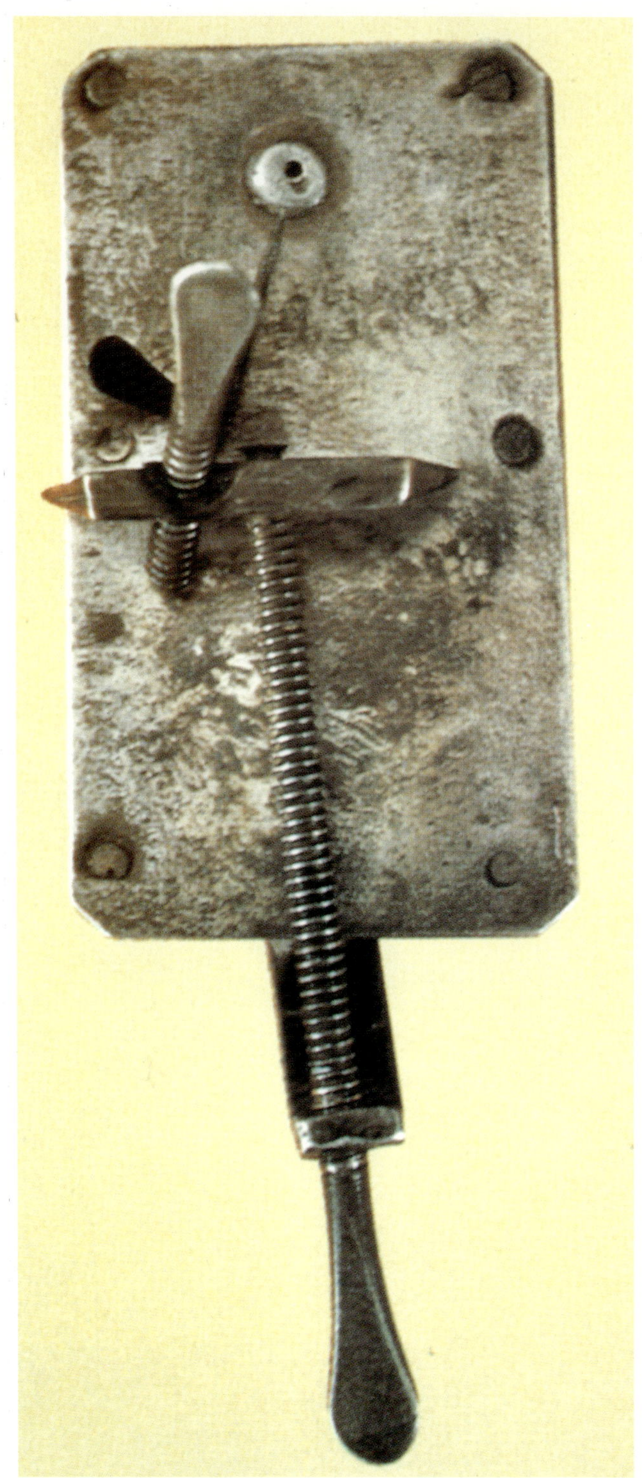

A modern replica of the prototype microscope built by Leeuwenhoek in about 1670. The specimen is mounted on the vertical spindle and viewed through the tiny lens at the top of the plate. The whole microscope is only the length of a matchbox.

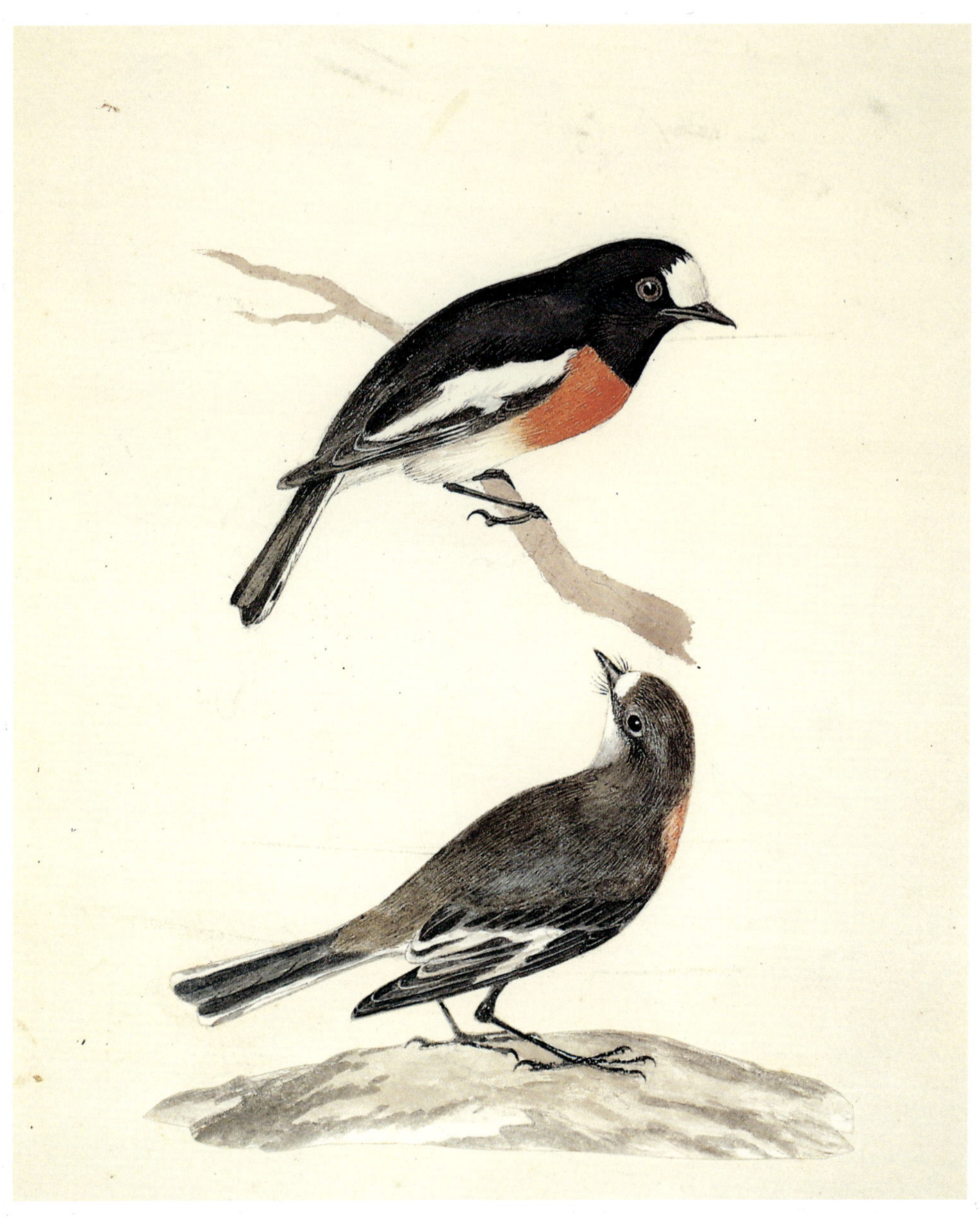

Recent scientific studies have shown that the brain centres responsible for song in birds grow dramatically before every breeding season. Black-throated Robin, *J. Cotton. La Trobe Library.*

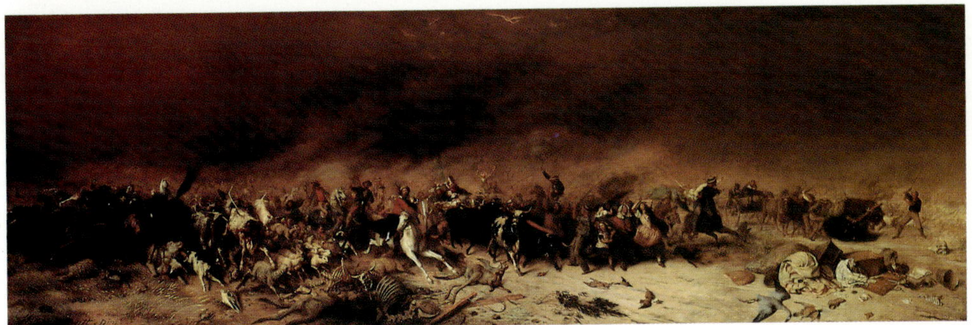

A bushfire spreads because it raises the temperature of surrounding vegetation above the combustion point. In much the same way, electrical activity spreads along a nerve because the action potential increases ion permeability in the adjacent area of the cell membrane and initiates another action potential. Black Thursday February 6th 1851, *W. Strutt. La Trobe Library.*

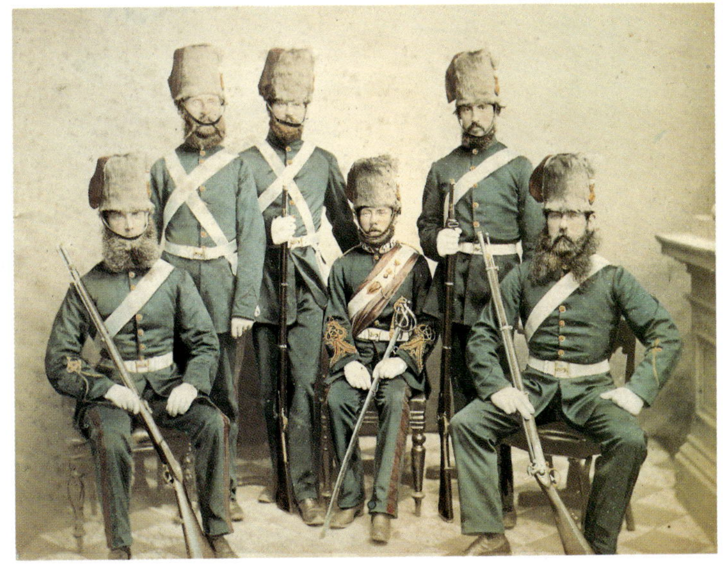

During the nineteenth century, many local militia groups like this company from Melbourne were set up in response to fears of war. In the body, circulating white blood cells have a similar, but more often called-on, role in guarding against infection. Richmond Volunteers' Regiment, *1861, Batchelor & O'Neil. La Trobe Library.*

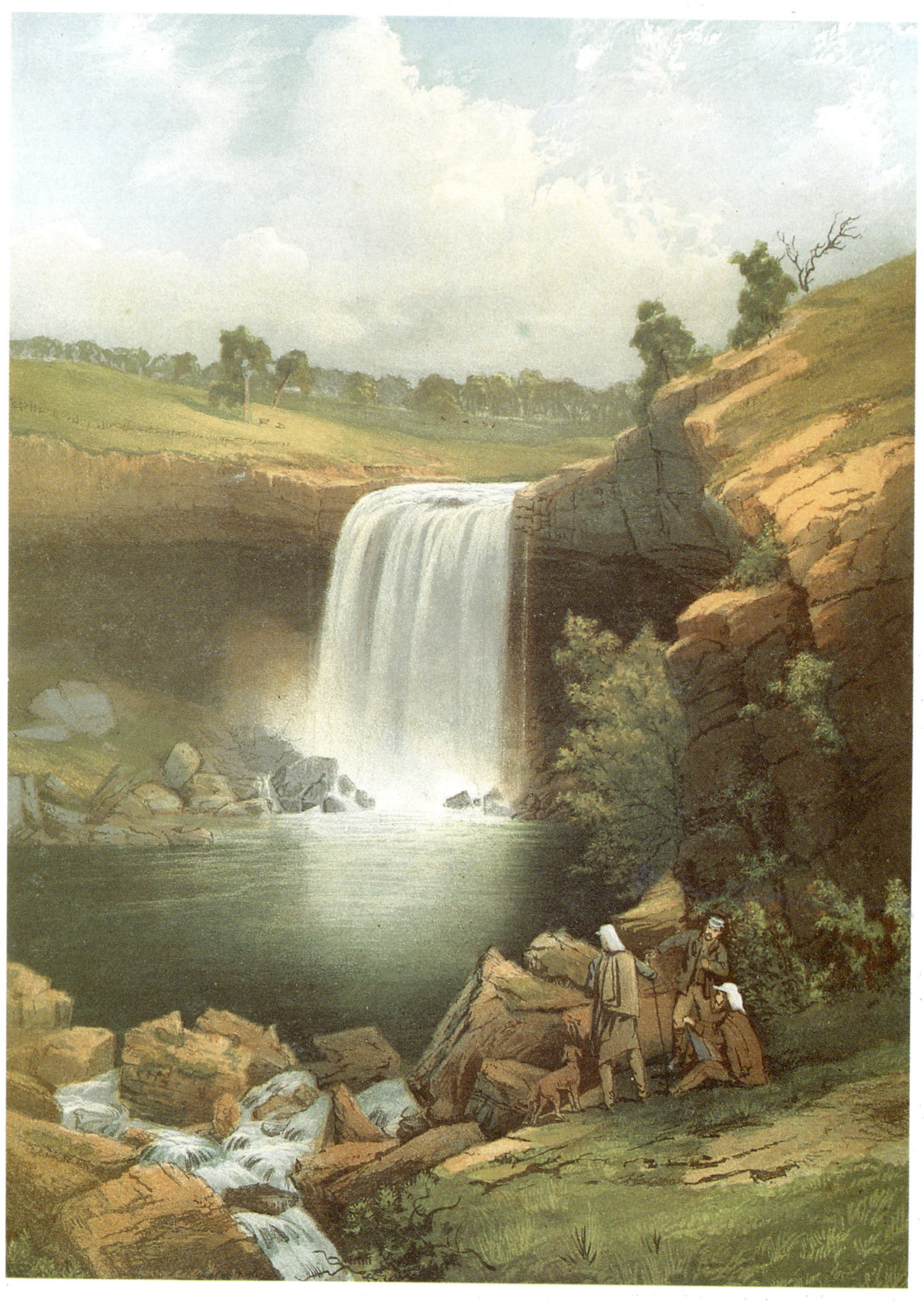

Just as with a waterfall, flow of blood from arteries to veins involves movement of fluid down a pressure gradient. Wannon Falls, *N. Chevalier. La Trobe Library.*

Each sodium ion carries a positive charge, further reducing the membrane voltage and so further increasing inward sodium movement: this corresponds to the paper bursting into flame. In the same way as the flame produced will also warm the surrounding paper, the loss of membrane voltage at one spot will slightly reduce voltage across adjacent areas of membrane, and cause the rapid inward sodium movement to spread. So a wave of sodium leakage, and consequent voltage change, travels along the whole length of the nerve. This is the action potential.

The speed at which nerve electricity is conducted is much less than the speed at which electricity moves in wires, so even the simplest sort of body reactions have a delay, or latency. When one picks up a hot object, it is dropped again in much less than a second, so action potentials must travel from the hand that is burnt to the brain, and back to the muscles that control hand movement (a total of about one metre) in this short a time. But you can also see that the reaction is not instantaneous, otherwise one would never get burnt!

Adding more efficient insulation to the outside of the nerve increases the speed at which action potentials move, and many of our nerves, including the ones that control movement, are coated with a fatty insulating substance called myelin. Some diseases, like multiple sclerosis, gradually destroy this layer of myelin, resulting in muscle weakness and paralysis.

So far we have talked about action potentials as though electricity flowed through the whole nervous system without any interruption. But, in fact, although an action potential can travel right along any one nerve cell, it cannot jump across the gap, or synapse, that separates adjacent cells. The functioning nervous system must therefore also use a second, quite different, process to enable information to be carried between cells. This process relies on the diffusion of a chemical messenger that is released by the action potential.

The ancients thought that the nerves worked as an interlinking system of tubes, through which the humours of the body flowed. Even last century, when biologists were first able to study the microscopic anatomy of the nervous system, it was accepted that all our nerves were one continuous unit. Two experimental findings overturned this view. The first was that particular dyes stained certain segments of the nervous system and left others unstained: the second was that the passage of information along some nerve pathways was possible only in one direction. These two observations established that the nervous system is made up of many quite separate cells, which must therefore have some means of conveying information from one to the other.

The way in which this information transfer occurs was the subject of a thirty-year controversy between the two greatest neurobiologists of this century. Henry Dale, who won the Nobel price in 1935, held the view that a chemical substance released from the ending of one nerve acted on the next nerve. John Eccles, who won the same prize in 1963, maintained that the action potential arriving at the terminal of one nerve produced a voltage change in the adjacent nerve without intervention of any chemical process. The matter was resolved only when measurement of the events inside a single nerve cell showed that the process that actually occurred could be explained only by the involvement of a chemical messenger.

How is the electrical activity of the action potential converted into chemical energy and back again? To understand this, we must first know something about the structural features of the region where the two nerves communicate: what we call the synaptic region. In the electron microscope, we can see that there is a very narrow gap (about one ten-thousandth of a millimetre) between the two cells, and that the ending of the cell bringing in information contains many small membrane-wrapped packets, or vesicles. These vesicles contain the chemical messenger substance.

The arrival of an action potential at the nerve ending causes some of the vesicles to fuse with the inside of the nerve surface, and to empty their messenger chemical into the gap between the cells. The messenger then diffuses across the gap, and locks into a specially shaped protein located on the second cell, in the same way as a key is inserted into a door lock. This process then opens holes in the surface membrane, just as turning the key in a lock opens the door. Positively charge ions rush through the holes into the cell, reducing the voltage difference between its inside and outside, and producing a new action potential.

Other types of nerve release chemical messengers that open different sized holes, and so allow different ions to move across the cell surface, thus increasing the voltage difference between the inside and outside. These nerves therefore stabilise the second cell, and prevent action potentials being produced. We could think of the action potential-producing nerves as 'excitatory' in function, and the stabilising nerves as 'inhibitory'. In many parts of the nervous system, both excitatory and inhibitory nerves are found.

The series of processes occurring at the synapse is very rapid, taking only about five-thousandths of a second. So during involuntary actions such as dropping a hot object, most of the delay is due to the time taken for action potentials to travel along the nerves, not for transfer of messages between them.

Muscle contraction, which is the final part of an involuntary action like this, involves another conversion of electrical into chemical energy. In this case, however, the chemical energy is itself converted into mechanical energy, and muscle movement results.

The contractions made by the various muscles in our bodies are essential for life in many ways. They provide rigidity for the skeleton, and allow us to walk, run and perform a myriad manipulative tasks. They also perform the work of breathing, provide the pressure needed to push blood around the body and move foodstuffs through the digestive tract.

Of course, the muscles that perform these very different tasks have some rather different properties, but they all have one thing in common – the microscopic structure by means of which they are able to shorten. This structure is called the sarcomere.

For many years it has been known that, under the microscope, most muscles have a crossbanded appearance, with alternating transverse stripes of dark and light material. The sets of stripes represent individual sarcomeres. In 1954 the English physiologist, Andrew Huxley, was able to show that when muscle contracted, the light stripes became narrower, while the dark stripes remained the same width. From this observation, Huxley realised that muscle contraction involves the sliding of longitudinally arranged strands past each other, rather than actual shortening of any tissue component. One set of strands, all lined up in

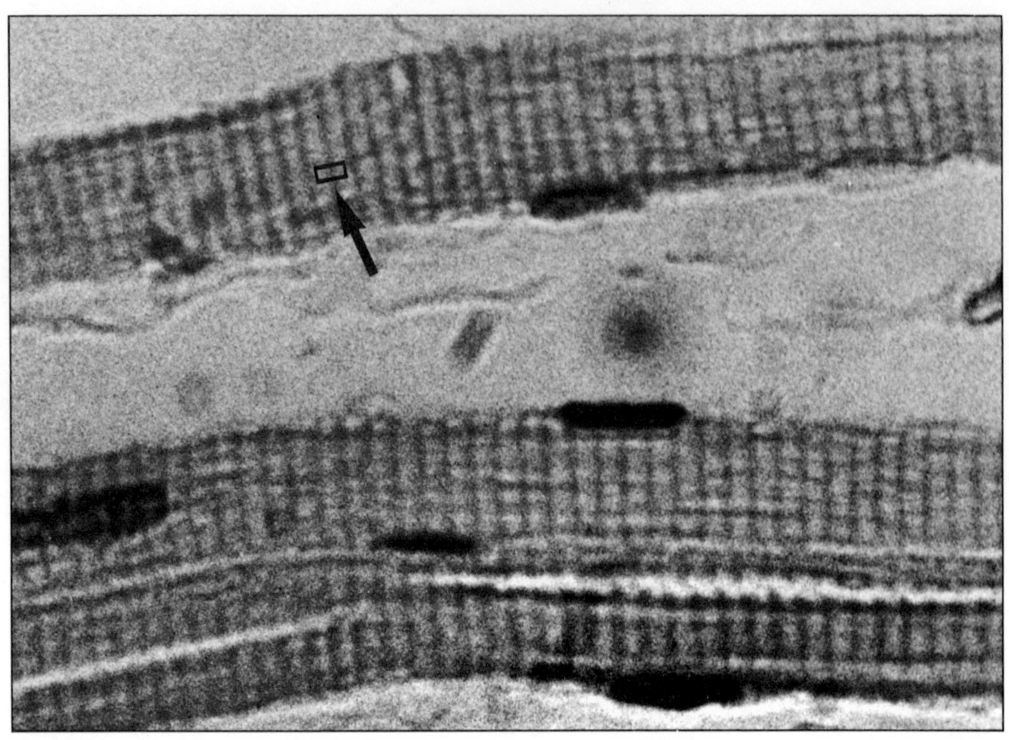

In a thin slice of muscle seen under the microscope, several long muscle cells stretch from left to right across this picture. Regular dark and light cross-bands can be seen along each cell. Huxley's discovery of the mechanism of muscle contraction stemmed from his observation that the distance between the dark bands shortened during the contraction. The portion of one muscle cell contained within the arrowed box is magnified in diagrammatic form in the next illustration.

parallel, could be seen as the dark stripes across the muscle. The other, lighter coloured strands slid past them during contraction. So while the distance between adjacent dark strands shrank, the length of the dark strands remained constant. You can see what Huxley was looking at if you hold a bundle of drinking straws in each hand, and slide them towards each other through a third bundle lying on the table. The straws you are holding are the light strands and the ones on the table are the dark strands. Your hands (the ends of the sarcomere) get closer together, but none of the straws actually change in length.

We now know a great deal about the processes that occur within a sarcomere during muscle contraction. The light strands are a protein called actin, and the dark strands another protein called myosin. Each myosin strand has many projecting sidearms along it, and the end of each sidearm contains an energy-storing substance called ATP. As well, each sidearm bears a specialised area like a key. Along each actin strand are rows of keyholes that will fit these keys, but when the muscle is resting these keyholes are covered over.

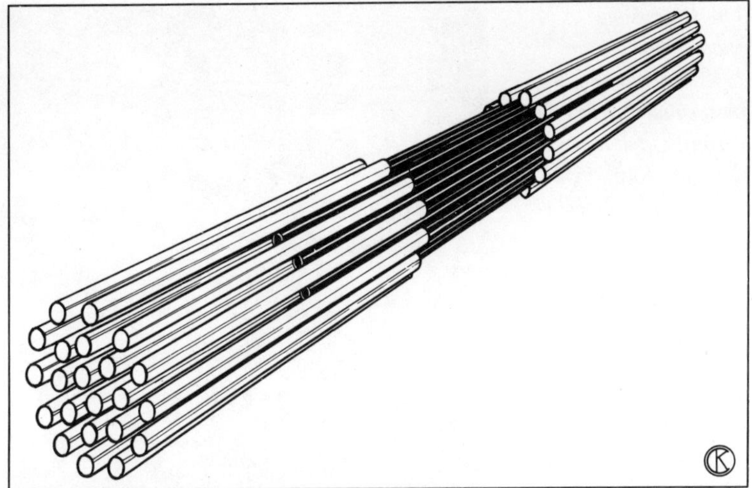

The cross-bands seen in muscle cells are made up of bundles of overlapping protein molecules which slide past each other during contraction, making the muscle shorter.

The occurrence of an action potential in the muscle cell causes the keyhole covers to be slid back, exposing the keyholes. Each of the myosin sidearm keys is then inserted into a keyhole. When this occurs, stored energy is freed from the ATP in the myosin sidearm, and this energy bends the sidearm and pushes the two strands past each other. Once movement of the sidearms has occurred, a new molecule of ATP replaces the original one that was in the sidearm. This removes the key from the keyhole, and separates the actin and myosin strands once again.

The muscle shortening that occurs with one interaction between myosin and actin moves the strands only a tiny distance past one another. Even the briefest contraction of a muscle in the body involves many repeated sequences of the same sort, rather like a row of men pulling in a rope. Also, remember that I have been talking about just one sarcomere. The whole muscle is made of thousands of these, arranged end to end, so the total amount of movement that occurs is much greater than in any one alone.

ATP, then, provides energy for two events in each actin-myosin interaction: the first is the movement, and the second is the disengagement of the myosin sidearm key from the actin keyhole, so it can be inserted into the next keyhole and more movement can occur. If the body is unable to make enough ATP to produce this disengagement, then the actin and myosin

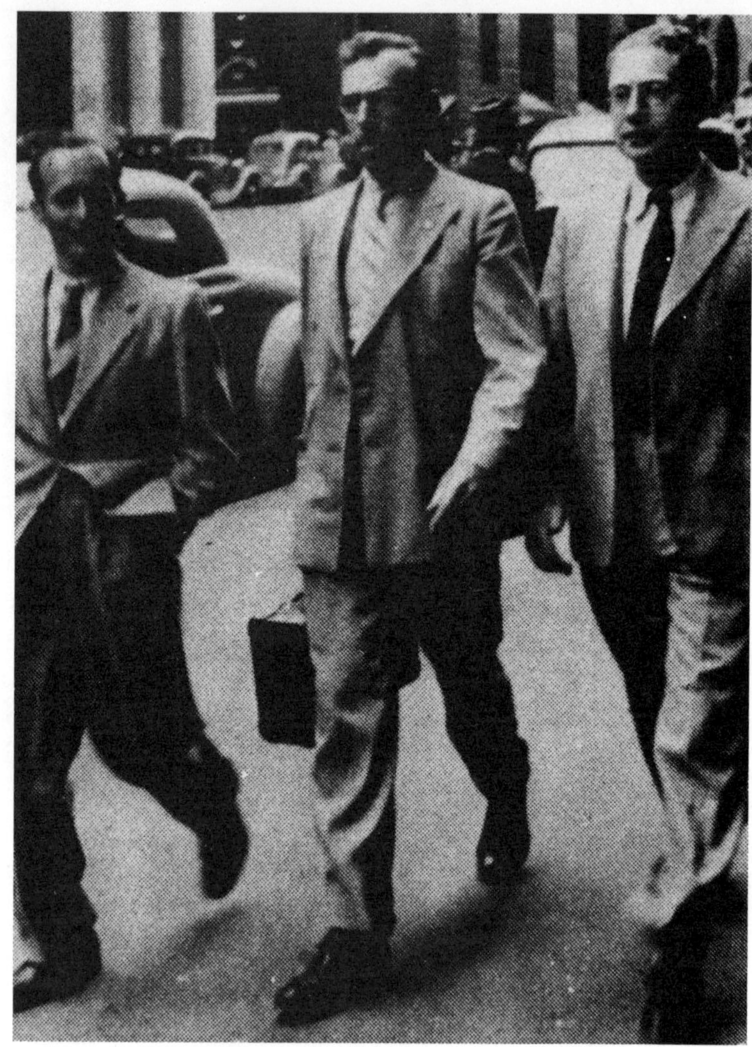

This remarkable photograph taken in 1940 shows three of the most eminent neuroscientists of all time. Bernhard Katz, on the right, won the Nobel prize in 1968 for his work on neurotransmission between nerves and muscle cells. John Eccles, in the centre, was awarded the same prize in 1963 for studies of neurotransmission in the spinal cord. On the left is Stephen Kuffler, whose main research involved the ways in which nerve cells adapt to different circumstances. At the time of this photograph, all three men were working at the Kanematsu Institute in Sydney Hospital.

remain locked together and the muscle is stiff. Here, then, is the explanation for the fact that bodies become rigid after death (rigor mortis).

The sequence of nerve and muscle events that produces muscle contraction still tells us hardly anything about the events that produce ordered movements of the body. These processes involve interactions between nerve cells that are much more complicated than those I have described so far, and include control of body functions like balance and blood circulation as well as muscle movements. We shall be looking at some aspects of these in later chapters.

THE ILLUMINATING SQUID

While human beings and other vertebrates move by using their limbs, some invertebrates use a totally different form of locomotion. The squid, for instance, swims by using the muscles of its body wall to squirt water out through a small hole. This produces a sort of jet propulsion. In view of this dramatic difference between species, it is intriguing that the crucial experimental work that led to an understanding of the processes of nerve conduction and communication between nerves and muscle cells was carried out almost completely using the squid.

The nerve fibres of mammals are so fine that until very recently it has not been practicable to measure events that take place inside them. But the nerves that supply the jet motor muscles of the squid are enormously thick, about a millimetre in diameter. To be effective, the squid's nerves have to conduct messages very rapidly. But invertebrates are not able to make the insulating substance myelin, which speeds up nerve conduction in mammals. However, conduction speed is also increased if the diameter of the nerve is larger. This alternative is possible for the squid because not many nerve fibres are needed to control the swimming muscles. It would not be possible for us because we would not be able to fit all our nerves into our bodies!

There were two experimental advantages of the 'giant' squid nerve. It was large enough for Cambridge scientists Hodgkin and Huxley to insert fine wires into it to directly measure electrical events associated with the action potential. As well, they were able to remove enough internal fluid from the nerve to show that its content of sodium was quite different from that outside. These unique properties of the squid axons are still used by biologists all over the world, to further understand the details of nerve behaviour.

Chapter Three

Blood is Richer than Water

Eight per cent of the weight of a human being is blood. This means that in most of us there is about five litres, or just over a gallon, of blood. If blood is allowed to stand so that it settles, or if this process is speeded up by centrifugation, it can be seen to consist of three components. A little more than half the total blood volume is fluid, the blood plasma, while almost all the rest consists of red and white blood cells. But between the light plasma and the heavier cells can be seen a tiny strip of another component, the platelets. Each of the three components has essential roles in keeping the body alive.

As well as containing large numbers of dissolved mineral particles such as sodium, potassium and calcium, and dissolved organic substances like the glucose needed for cell nourishment, the plasma also contains three types of dissolved proteins, each with a specific and independent function. The most abundant of these proteins is albumin, very similar in structure to the albumin that makes up egg white. The albumin molecules attract water around them and so prevent it leaking out of the blood stream into the tissues. Without this, it would not be possible to maintain sufficient plasma volume to keep the blood cells in circulation.

The next most abundant proteins are a group known as the globulins. Some globulins are able to bind onto various hormones, and serve to carry these in the bloodstream. Others, the immunoglobulins, are the sites of protective antibodies against infections. The third, and least abundant, type of protein is called fibrinogen, and forms the fibrous meshwork that produces a blood clot when bleeding occurs.

The cells present in blood originate from the marrow that forms the core of the bones. Red and white cells and platelets are

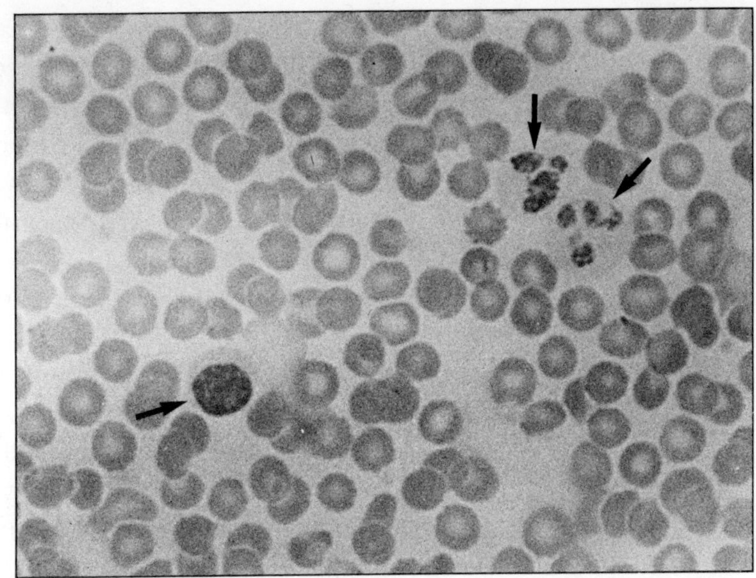

A smear of blood can be seen to contain several different sorts of cells. The smallest and most numerous are the red cells that carry oxygen. The others (arrowed) are different varieties of white cells, concerned with fighting infection.

all produced from the same population of marrow cells, but, as they mature, they become specialised in different ways.

The red blood cells, or erythrocytes, are dedicated to carrying oxygen and carbon dioxide between the lungs and all the cells of the body. In order to perform this task, the erythrocyte changes as it grows from a sphere into a doughnut shape. This increases its surface area and makes gas diffusion in and out of the cell more efficient. It also makes the erythrocyte flexible, so that it can be squeezed through the narrow capillaries where gas exchange occurs.

Another specialised feature of the erythrocyte is its content of the protein haemoglobin, which is necessary for carrying oxygen. In fact, about one-third of the total weight of a red blood cell is haemoglobin. Even tiny alterations in the structure of this molecule have dramatic effects on its capacity to carry oxygen. So any mutation in the genetic blueprint for haemoglobin can result in defects in red cell function, or anaemia. One of the most common of these genetic defects is a serious health problem in a geographic belt that stretches all the way from the Mediterranean to Thailand, causing a profound anaemia that is known as thalassaemia.

Apart from the genetic requirements for satisfactory formation of haemoglobin, three dietary factors are also essential for red cell production and the prevention of anaemia. Two of these are vitamin B_{12} and folic acid, which are needed to enable the cells to mature normally. Folic acid is present in many foodstuffs, but appreciable amounts of vitamin B_{12} are found only in products of animal origin. It is therefore wise for vegetarians to have a regular intake of cheese or eggs, to ensure that they receive adequate supplies of this vitamin.

The third essential dietary factor is iron, which forms part of the haemoglobin molecule. Many foods contain abundant iron, but the amount that is absorbed through the intestine depends very much on the type of food eaten. Iron in meat, which is already bound to haemoglobin, is absorbed easily, but the iron in cereals is hardly absorbed at all because of the presence of certain other substances. So, once again, vegetarians develop anaemia more easily than other people, and must be particularly careful in planning a balanced diet.

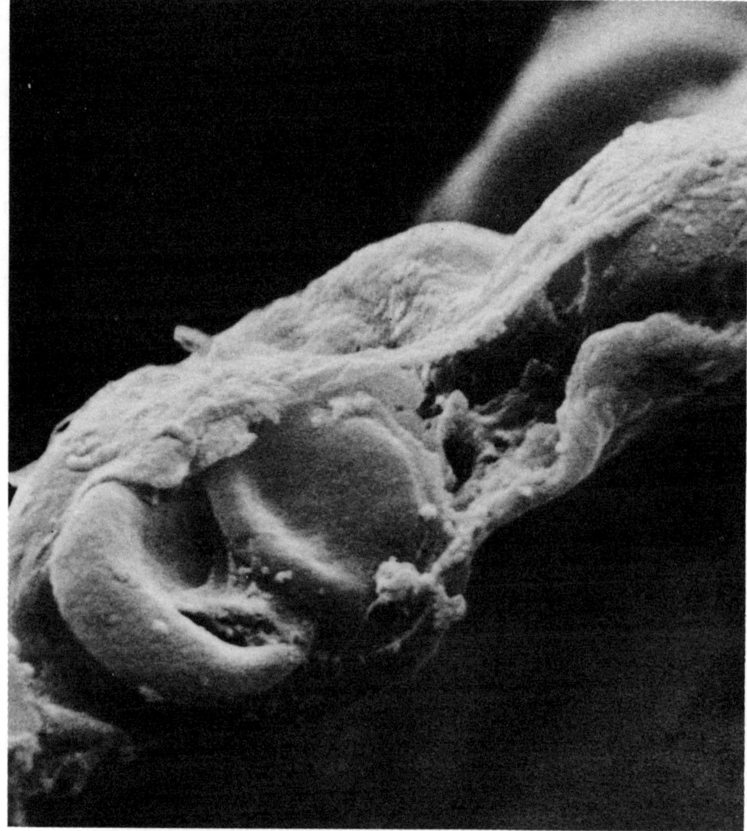

Red blood cells are highly specialised for their job of carrying oxygen to the body's tissues. Their doughnut shape provides a large surface area for gas diffusion, and allows them to squeeze through the small capillaries where gas exchange occurs. Here, the scanning electron microscope reveals two blood cells passing along a capillary.

Because red blood cells take a long time to grow, and because they play a crucial role in carrying oxygen around the body, it is essential to have efficient ways in which the loss of blood can be minimised after damage to a blood vessel. The process by which bleeding is stopped, haemostasis, is triggered by the tiny platelets in the blood stream. These platelets stick to most tissue surfaces that they contact, with the exception of the thin layer of specialised cells that line all blood vessels. So, if the underlying layers of the vessel wall are exposed, platelets rapidly stick to the damaged area, forming a plug that will close any small leak.

As the platelets collect, they also release a number of powerful chemical substances that help in the haemostatic process. Some of these chemicals contract the muscle cells in the vessel wall, shutting off the further flow of blood. Others take part in the final, and slowest, component of haemostasis: the formation of the blood clot.

Damage to the vessel lining not only causes aggregation of platelets, but also triggers a crucial structural change in a plasma protein called Factor 12. This transforms the protein from a biologically inert molecule into an active one, capable of recognising and attacking another particular protein present in the plasma. In turn, this process activates the second protein so it can attack a third, and the third a fourth. Each of these recognition steps can occur only in the vicinity of the platelet-derived chemicals.

The proteins in this chain of events are collectively called 'clotting factors', and a total of about a dozen are involved. Once it is started, the activation of successive factors progresses automatically, just as a row of standing dominoes collapses progressively when one is pushed. The final link in the chain is a long, thread-like molecule called fibrin. When activated, the fibrin molecules all stick together, forming a meshwork. This surrounds the platelet plug, ensnares neighbouring blood cells and blocks off the site of blood vessel damage completely. Viewed through an electron microscope, the blood clot at this stage looks rather like a bowl of spaghetti and meat balls.

Over the next few hours, the clot becomes more and more solid, as further chemical reactions take place. At the same time, however, a much slower process of reversal has begun. The very protein factor that initiated the sequence of clot formation also activated a blood protein with the ability to gradually dissolve the fibrin threads. By the time that the processes of tissue repair have mended the damaged vessel wall, the clot will have started to disintegrate, so that normal blood flow can be restored.

Because the clotting process is triggered by contact of the blood with damaged tissue, clot formation usually only occurs at these sites. By this reasoning, it might be assumed that blood that is withdrawn directly into a glass container would not clot. However, the truth is that clotting occurs at nearly the same rate in either situation. In fact, contact with glass or metal surfaces activates the clotting sequence just as contact with damaged tissues does. To minimise this, glass containers used for handling blood are lubricated inside with silicone, so that they resemble the lining of an intact blood vessel.

Sometimes a clot formed inside a damaged vessel is dislodged before it has been broken down, and is carried along by the bloodstream. Usually these free-floating clots, or thrombi, are

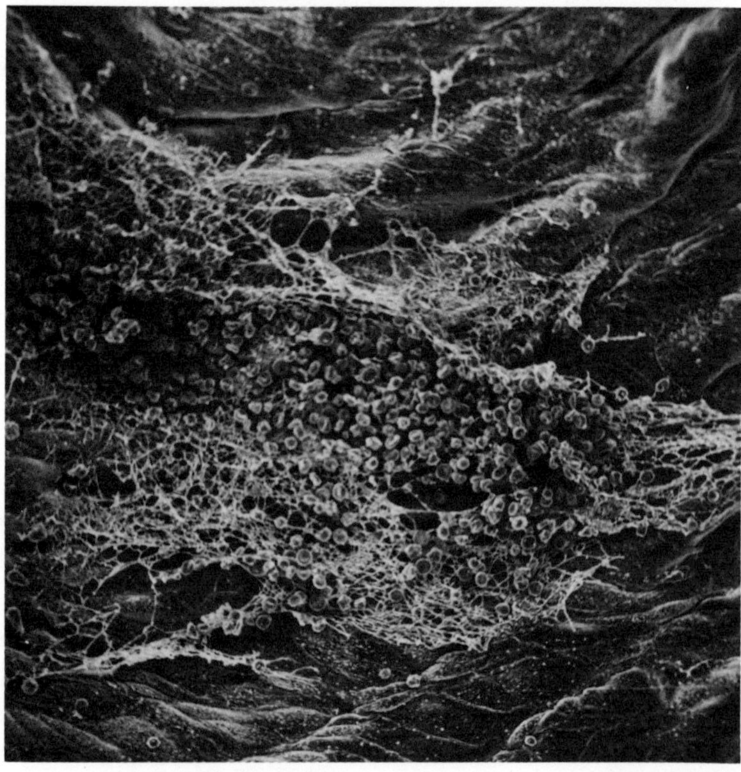

A blood clot consists of blood cells, trapped in a sticky mesh of fibrin molecules.

trapped and destroyed in the vessels of the lung, which contains large amounts of clot-dissolving enzymes. But, very occasionally, a clot escapes into the arterial circulation. Here, it may block the blood supply to part of an important organ such as the heart, causing a heart attack, or the brain, causing a stroke. The rareness of such events, however, emphasises how precisely the factors that stimulate and inhibit haemostasis interact with each other.

While the red blood cells have the specialised task of providing oxygen and removing carbon dioxide, the white blood cells, or leucocytes, are specialised for an entirely different task – that of defending the body against invasion by foreign organisms. The processes that make up these defences are known collectively as immunity.

Immunologists distinguish many separate types of white cell, but in broad terms they can be divided into three groups on the basis of the ways in which they attack an invading microbe. These are by the production of antibodies, by secretion of biologically active chemicals, and by physically attacking the invader.

One large group of white cells, called lymphocytes, are trained to recognise particular proteins and sugars on the microbe's surface. They respond to these by manufacturing specialised globulin molecules, or antibodies, which they secrete into the bloodstream. The antibodies then stick to the component of the microbe that they recognise. Because antibodies produced in response to different microbes are slightly different in shape, each of them will only stick to that particular sort of microbe, in the same way that keys and locks are matched individually.

Antibody production takes up to several weeks, but after one exposure to a particular microbe, the lymphocytes usually store a memory of the process. So if a second infection with the same organism occurs, antibodies can be made much more quickly than on the first occasion. This is the basis of immunisation against infections like polio, tetanus and diphtheria, where the microbe is pretreated to make it less dangerous and then injected. The lymphocytes remember some microbes for many years, but forget some others, like the cholera bacterium, quite rapidly. So immunisation against cholera is only effective for a few months. A few viruses, like the one that causes the common cold, seem to be forgotten almost immediately, and we never develop resistance to them.

The process of tagging a specific antibody to a microbe triggers the successive activation of a series of plasma proteins, rather like the sequence involved in blood clotting. In this case, however, the final active proteins that are produced, which are called 'complement', are able to attach to the tagged microbe, destroy its outer membrane, and kill it. Although the antibody is needed for recognition of a foreign cell, therefore, it does not actually do the job of repelling the invader.

The effectiveness of this system for prevention of infections obviously depends entirely on the ability of the lymphocytes to correctly identify particular microbes. Unfortunately, the identification process can be disrupted in the presence of certain viruses, with the result that antibodies are not produced in response to invasion by other, dangerous microbes. The danger of this sort of 'acquired' immune deficiency syndrome (AIDS) is therefore not the infection by the AIDS virus itself, but loss of resistance to other infections such as pneumonia.

As well as attack by complement, there are two other ways in which the immune system destroys invading cells. One of these involves the physical absorption of the foreign organism into a specialised type of white cell, with its subsequent digestion. The second, which is especially important in fighting viral infections, involves a protein called interferon.

Viruses lack the cellular machinery that is normally used for energy production, and they can multiply in the body only by entering a cell and converting its machinery to their own purposes. Once inside the cell, the virus is protected from most of the body's immune defences. Interferon, however, stimulates the cell to manufacture new substances that inhibit viral activity. As well, interferon mobilises a specialised group of lymphocytes which are capable of recognising and destroying the particular cells in which the virus is hiding.

This last property has recently been the subject of intense research interest, because the lymphocytes can recognise not only virus-containing cells, but also other abnormal cells such as cancer cells. It is therefore likely that they function as a continual surveillance system, ensuring that tiny cancers are destroyed before they become large enough to be dangerous. Unfortunately, it is all too clear that this system is not foolproof. But the possibility exists that some cancers develop only because there is insufficient interferon production in the body. In these cases, treatment with interferon may have dramatic effects.

ANAEMIA

Anaemia is any state where the haemoglobin of the red blood cells is insufficient to carry as much oxygen as the body needs. The reduced haemoglobin can be due to any of a number of factors, but most cases of anaemia result from its production being defective.

This haemoglobin deficiency may occur because the bone marrow is not able to produce blood cells, as a result of exposure to irradiation or to certain chemicals. A second cause of insufficient cell production is a lack of one of the dietary factors needed for red cell growth: vitamin B_{12}, or folate, or iron. Thirdly, the haemoglobin molecule itself may be abnormal, because of a genetic defect.

The thalassaemias that were mentioned in the text of this chapter are the most common disorder of this type, and, in fact, are one of the most common genetic disorders in the world. The lifelong anaemia that they cause is a considerable long term health problem in the affected populations, because there is no effective treatment except frequent blood transfusion. Fortunately, it is possible to recognise carriers of the defective gene, and to identify the presence of thalassaemia in samples of foetal blood. Preventive programmes based on these techniques are now being instituted in Sardinia, Greece and other places where the incidence of this fatal disease is highest.

A second hereditary defect occurs mainly in populations of Negro descent. Here the haemoglobin molecule responds

The hereditary anaemic disease thalassaemia occurs commonly in the areas of the world shaded on the map.

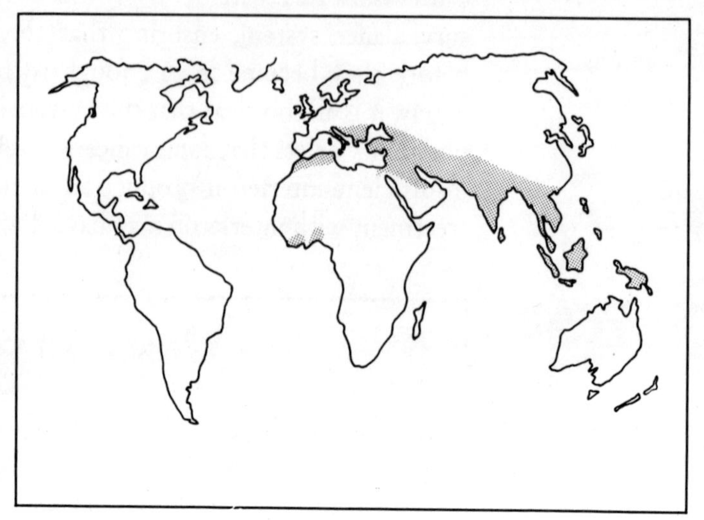

abnormally to changes in local oxygen concentration, becoming physically distorted when the amount of oxygen falls. This has an effect on the red blood cells rather like putting a coat hanger inside a balloon: the cells become fragile and lose the flexibility that normally allows them to squeeze through the smallest blood vessels. Unlike thalassaemia, this so-called sickle cell anaemia is often free of severe ill-effects. But, if an affected person is exposed to low oxygen concentrations, for instance at high altitude, then the distorted blood cells are likely to block blood flow through some vessels and cause tissue damage.

Most genetic defects seem to be wholly without use to the body. However, the genes that produce thalassaemia and sickle cell disease both make the bearer resistant to infection by the malaria parasite. So, in the areas of the world where these mutations originated, they may actually have been beneficial rather than harmful.

Chapter Four

Staying in Circulation

Blood flowing through the capillaries continually conveys essential foodstuffs and oxygen to all cells of the body, and collects from them waste products such as lactic acid and carbon dioxide. Liquids will flow only from regions of high to regions of lower pressure. So for blood to flow around the body, there must be a pressure gradient between arteries and veins. This is generated by the pressure produced inside the heart when it beats.

Most hydraulic pumps produce a continuous outflow of liquid, but as the pumping contractions of the heart are separated by the relaxation periods that are needed to refill the ventricles, blood flow out of the heart is only intermittent. However, exchange of wastes and nutrients across the capillary wall is most efficient when flow through the capillaries is continuous. So, to achieve this, there must be mechanisms by which the pulsatile cardiac ejection is converted into a steady stream.

Two mechanisms are involved. The first of these is the existence of a large resistance to flow through the arterial system upstream of the capillaries. As the arteries branch and become smaller and smaller in diameter, their resistance to flow increases. This slows the rate at which blood can leave the arterial system, in the same way as reducing the diameter of a garden hose by standing on it slows the water flow out the end. Blood movement from the arteries into the capillaries therefore still continues after the end of each heart beat.

Even so, if the blood vessels were rigid tubes (like a garden hose is) then heart rate would have to be very high to keep capillary perfusion (the flow of blood through the capillaries) constant. However, they are not rigid. That part of the arterial system nearest to the heart, the aorta, has quite elastic walls, so

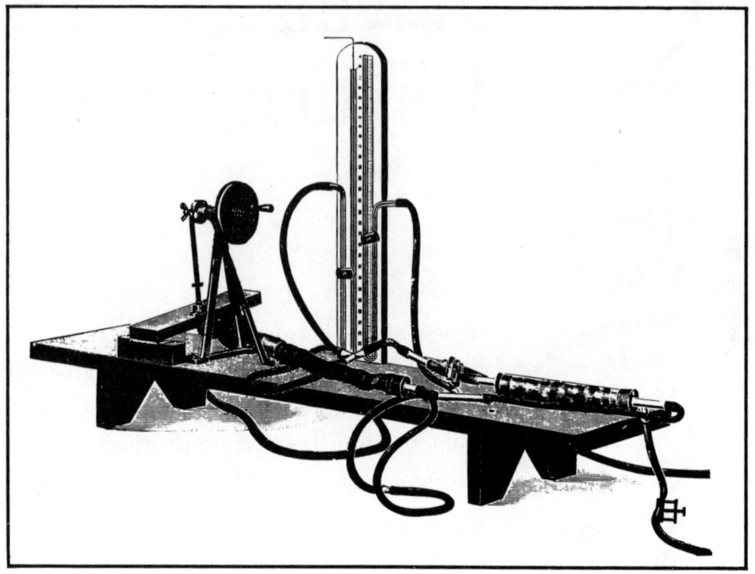

The system of heart and blood vessels responsible for carrying blood around the body has many similarities to a rubber bulb and a system of rubber tubes. This model was built in about 1900 to teach medical students the basic properties of the circulation. The heart is worked by turning the wheel on the left, and pressures at various points around the circuit are measured from the heights of columns of fluid in the U-tubes. An adjustable screw clamp, representing the arterial resistance, can be seen. Similar models to this are still used as teaching aids for students of physiology.

that pressure produced by cardiac ejection not only pushes blood forward but also increases aortic volume. In between beats, the stretched aortic walls contract again, and this continues to push the blood along, just as when you let go an inflated balloon the air is pushed out and makes the balloon fly around the room.

The pressure within that section of the arterial system upstream of the small, high-resistance vessels is what we monitor as blood pressure. It is typically expressed in terms of a higher and a lower value, for instance 120 on 80, or 120/80, millimetres of mercury. The higher, or systolic, pressure corresponds to the maximum pressure that is produced when the heart contracts, and the lower, or diastolic, value is the level to which pressure falls between heart beats.

As some of the energy of cardiac ejection is used to expand the aorta, the absolute value of systolic blood pressure will depend on aortic elasticity. The elastic components of the aortic wall deteriorate with age, so as we grow older, there is characteristically an increase in systolic pressure. Conversely, certain connective tissue diseases increase aortic elasticity. In these patients, during cardiac ejection, a part of the aorta may blow out into an aortic aneurysm.

While systolic pressure is affected by how much the arteries can stretch, diastolic pressure depends primarily on arterial resistance. This resistance is normally regulated by the amount of contraction of the muscle cells in the arterial walls. Contraction is produced both by circulating hormones and by the release of the neurotransmitter, noradrenaline, from nerve fibres around the vessels.

An abnormally high peripheral resistance to flow, and the consequent high diastolic pressure, is characteristic of high blood pressure, or hypertension. Most of the medicines that are prescribed to treat hypertension act by reducing flow resistance, although some are effective because they reduce the volume of blood that has to be pumped around the body.

Expenditure on medical treatment for hypertension makes

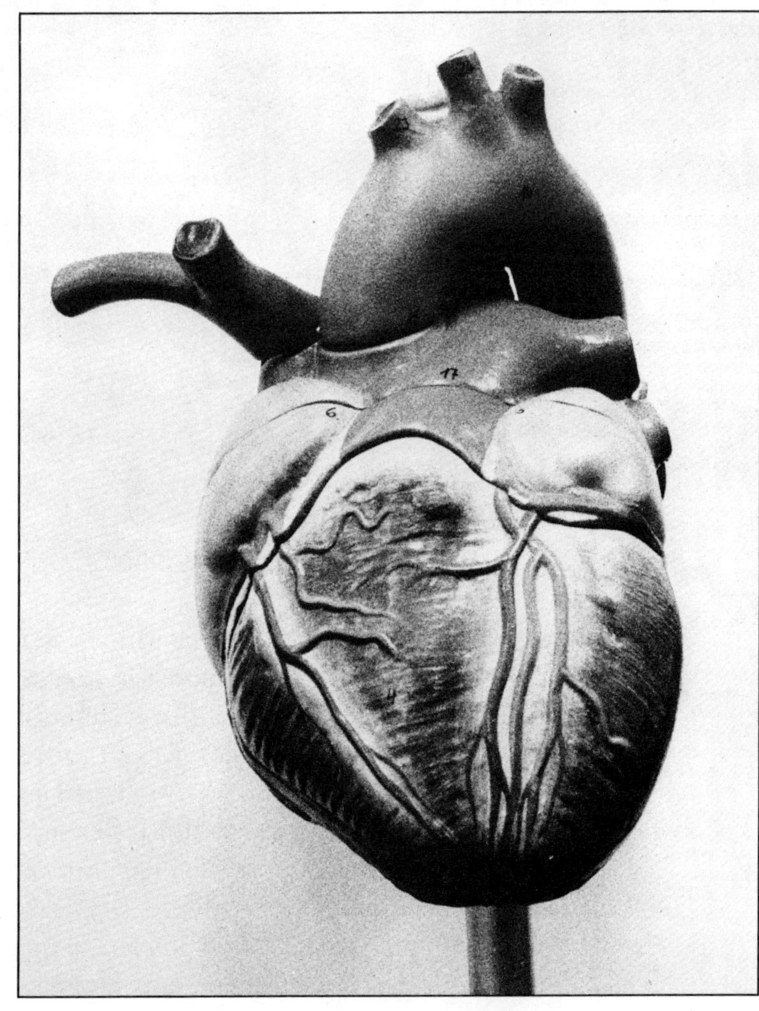

The blood supply essential to nourish the muscle of the heart itself travels in a network of coronary arteries, here seen running across the surface of a model heart.

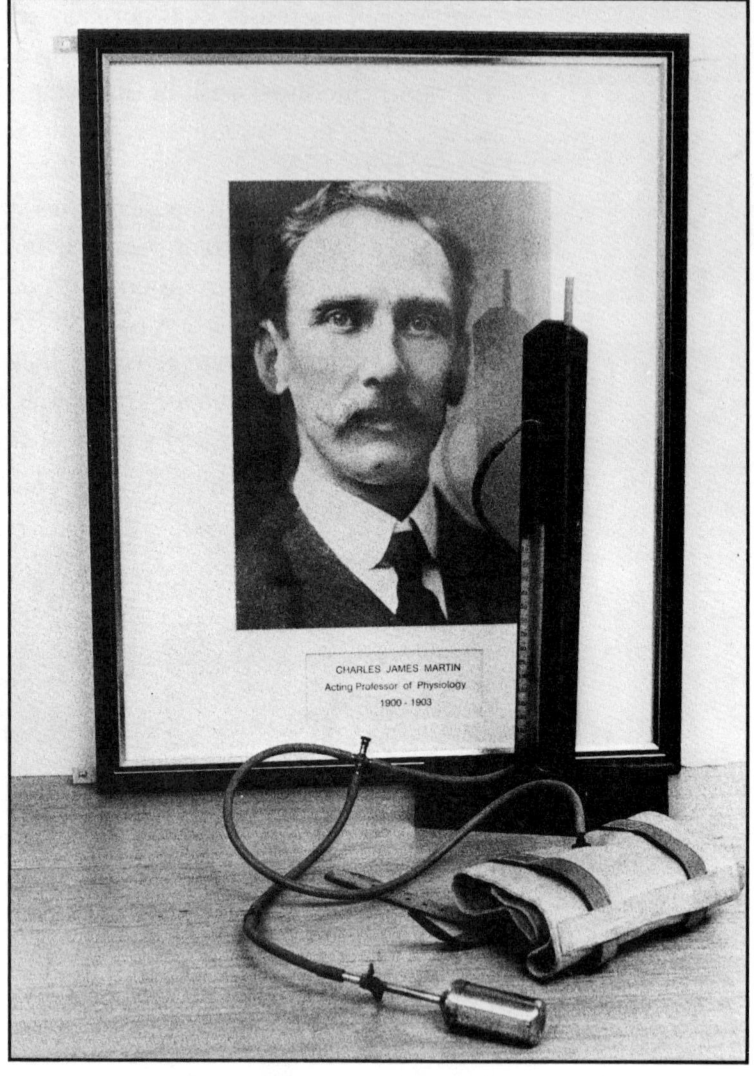

The sphygmomanometer that doctors routinely use to measure blood pressure was invented in 1896 by Scipione Riva Rocci. This more accurate and portable version was developed in the Physiology Department at Melbourne University by Professor Charles Martin in about 1900, and sold widely in Australia. It was priced at 25 shillings, and a wooden case was available at half a crown extra.

up a sizeable segment of the national health budget. A cheaper and more satisfactory approach would be to prevent blood pressure rising in the first place. Unfortunately, in the majority of cases, very little is known about the process, except that the normal control pathways are altered in some way. There is evidence for involvement of many factors, including salt intake, obesity, and changes in the brain, but the ways in which these interact in particular individuals is far from clear. Further research into the way blood pressure is controlled is therefore of great importance for community health.

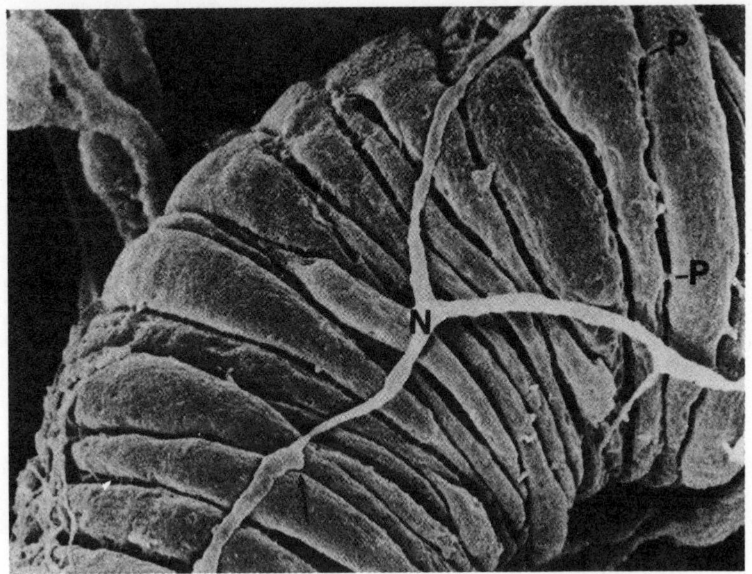

In this electron microscope view of a small artery, the muscle cells are seen to coil around the vessel, making it easy to understand how muscle contraction is able to shrink the arterial diameter. A single nerve axon (N), responsible for controlling vessel contraction, snakes over the muscle surface.

The continual flow of blood through the capillaries that is produced by cardiac pumping is essential for the nutrition of all the tissues in the body, but in the event that this flow falls, the brain is by far the most easily damaged organ. This is because the nerve cells of the brain are exceptionally sensitive to changes in oxygen supply. A substantial fall in blood flow to the brain for more than a few seconds inevitably causes loss of consciousness. So, it is essential for survival that some mechanisms exist to keep blood pressure, and therefore brain blood flow, fairly constant.

For animals like humans that stand on their hindlegs, there is a continual and serious difficulty in maintaining a stable blood pressure – the effect of gravity. Most of us have had the experience of feeling dizzy when we stand up suddenly after lying down. It is especially likely to have happened when one has been lying in the sun, or in a hot bath. When we stand up, the blood travelling from our hearts to our feet and back again becomes two continuous vertical columns of liquid. This increases the pressure inside the blood vessels of the legs and feet, and so blood accumulates in the easily stretched veins of the legs. The consequence is that less blood gets back to the heart, less is available to be pumped out, and blood pressure falls. The dizziness on standing results from the sudden lack of oxygen to the brain, and this effect is most noticeable when we are hot, because heat relaxes the vein walls and allows them to trap more blood.

However, people do not usually get dizzy when they stand up, and any faintness lasts only for a few moments, demonstrating that very efficient compensatory mechanisms exist. The most important of these is a system of neural pathways called the baroreceptor reflex.

In the walls of the arteries supplying blood to the head, there are nerve endings that monitor how much the arterial walls are stretched. If blood pressure falls, the wall is less stretched, and the firing rate of the nerves drops. This information is carried to a group of cells in the base of the brain, which functions as a control centre for blood pressure. The control centre is preset to maintain pressure at a particular level, much as a thermostat regulates temperature in an oven. Detection of a pressure fall activates other nerves that supply the heart and the muscle cells of the arteries, causing heart rate to increase and arterial resistance to rise. Together, these reflex responses restore blood pressure towards its previous level.

The nervous system compensations for reduced blood pressure when we stand up are usually assisted by contraction of the muscles responsible for leg movement. The leg veins have numerous one-way valves in them that allow blood to flow only towards the heart, like those in the veins of the arm that were seen by Harvey and used as evidence for his theory of blood circulation (see Chapter 1). Venous compression by the contracting leg muscles therefore squeezes the pooled blood out of the legs, and increases the amount available for cardiac ejection.

When this mechanical assistance of venous return is not available, the baroreceptor reflex alone may not be sufficient to guarantee adequate brain blood flow. So, for instance, soldiers standing to attention, and therefore not moving their leg muscles, sometimes faint on parade in hot weather. A more extreme situation is that experienced by test pilots and astronauts, who are subjected to very large gravitational forces. In order to retain consciousness, these individuals have to wear tight elastic clothing (G-suits) that restricts the volume of their bodies below heart level.

When we are upright, the extra pressure in the blood vessels

When a person stands motionless, blood tends to pool in the veins of the legs. Sometimes, this can reduce the amount returning to the heart so much that blood pressure falls dramatically, and the person faints.

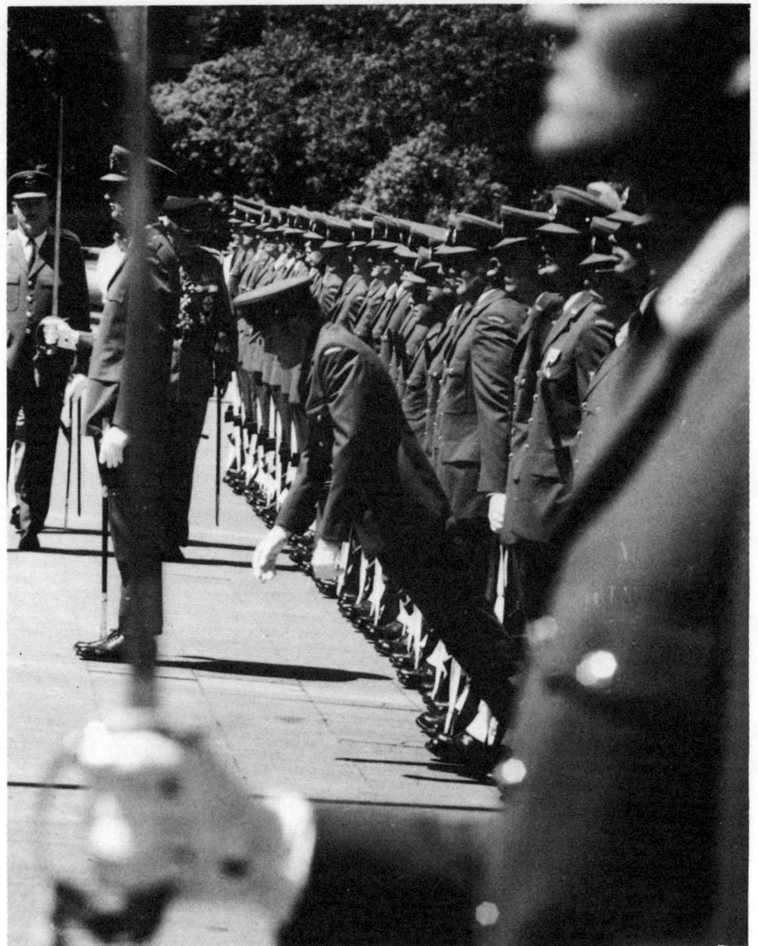

of the legs produces another problem as well as that of lowered venous return. Water molecules are forced out through the walls of the capillary vessels, causing uncomfortable tissue oedema. Usually, this swelling is minimal because contractions of the leg muscles compress the vessels, reducing the pressure difference across their walls and reducing the weight of blood present. On the other hand, when one is relatively immobile for a long time, for instance in an aeroplane or when serving in a shop, the leg muscles are not working, and so one's feet and ankles swell.

While the cells of the brain require a constant blood supply, most other groups of cells in the body have very variable demands for blood at various times, depending on their rate of consumption of oxygen and foodstuffs. For instance, the amount of blood needed by muscles during exercise is very much greater than the amount that the same tissues need when resting. This means that, as well as physiological mechanisms for controlling total peripheral resistance and blood pressure, the body must have mechanisms by which flow to particular organs can be controlled. While the control of blood pressure is mediated primarily through neural pathways, control of regional blood flow is mainly by local phenomena.

Because the circulation is responsible for removal of metabolic waste products from tissues as well as for the supply of nourishment, a fall in blood flow will cause accumulation of these wastes, or metabolites, around the vessels. The presence of metabolites is recognised chemically by the cells of the vessel walls, probably by means of receptor proteins like those involved at nerve synapses, and the vessels respond by relaxing and reducing the resistance to flow. If the rate of tissue activity rises, as occurs in muscles during exercise, then the rate of metabolite accumulation also rises, so local blood flow increases. When the muscles stop working, the extra wastes are quickly washed away, the blood vessels contract again and blood flow falls back to normal.

It is easy to see this relationship between tissue metabolism and blood flow by using a home blood pressure kit. When the cuff is placed on one arm and kept at a pressure well above the systolic blood pressure – so no blood flows through that forearm – metabolites build up and the blood vessels relax. If the cuff is released after about two minutes, the low vascular resistance will cause increased blood flow, which can be seen as flushing when you compare the colours of both arms.

The waste products of cellular activity not only relax blood vessels, but also stimulate nerve endings that carry pain information. This can be confirmed by contracting the forearm muscles while the blood pressure cuff is blown up. The rapid build-up of metabolites causes tingling and aching of the arm. Some disease processes change the properties of the arterial walls so that they cannot relax fully in response to local metabolites, and if this happens then increased tissue activity causes pain. The coronary arteries that supply blood to the muscle of the heart are particularly susceptible to this. When the increased demand of the heart muscle for blood during exercise is not matched by increased blood flow, the pain caused by metabolite accumulation is known as angina.

Movement of waste products and of nutrients between the bloodstream and the cells outside occurs through the walls of the capillaries. Each capillary is just wide enough for blood cells to squeeze through in single file, and the walls are only about half a micrometre thick, or about one hundred times thinner than a human hair.

Molecules move across the walls of the capillaries by diffusing from regions of high to low concentration. In most tissues, quite large substances such as proteins can move across the capillary wall, and in some, such as in bone marrow, there are gaps in the wall large enough for whole blood cells to penetrate. In the brain, however, the capillary walls are permeable only to very small molecules, and form what is known as the blood-brain barrier. The presence of this barrier means that medicines intended for use within the brain must be specially designed, although it also has the advantage that substances can be given to treat peripheral diseases without affecting the brain.

Capillary permeability not only varies from tissue to tissue but can be increased by a variety of local hormones, such as histamine and small protein fragments called kinins. These substances are released from injured tissue, and play a vital part in the resistance of the body to infection. The increased permeability allows antibodies and white blood cells to move out from the bloodstream into the damaged area, destroying invading bacteria and removing cellular debris. Water, too, moves out through the capillary wall, producing the tissue swelling that is characteristic of most injuries. The processes of repair are enhanced by the fact that the same local hormones that affect capillary permeability also relax the vascular muscle cells. So there is an increased local blood flow, bringing more white cells to the area of damage and, typically, making the area appear flushed.

Interestingly, the very same substances that are released from damaged cells are also present in stinging nettles and insect venoms. The local swelling that these stings cause is therefore also due to leakage of fluid out of the capillaries.

WHAT ARE 'HEART ATTACKS'?

When one of the small arteries that carry blood to the muscle of the heart is blocked, this portion of the heart is deprived of oxygen. The lack of oxygen and the accumulation of cell waste products are detected by the nervous system as pain (angina). If blood flow is stopped for long enough, the muscle cells in this part of the heart stop contracting and the heart's ability to pump blood is reduced. This reduces blood flow to the brain, so the victim may faint.

The most common reason for blockage of the coronary arteries is the build-up of fatty material on the inner wall of the vessel. If this is slight, then blood flow to the heart is only prejudiced when the heart is working extra hard. So attacks of angina occur during exercise but not at rest.

More rarely, a coronary artery shuts down without there being any physical blockage. Researchers are still trying to find the mechanisms that cause this sort of heart attack.

WHAT IS 'HIGH BLOOD PRESSURE'?

Blood pressure depends mainly on the amount of resistance to blood flow in the blood vessels. So, if the diameters of the vessels are reduced, pressure rises, just as the pressure in a hose rises if you stand on it while the water is running. Blood pressure varies quite a lot from person to person, and depends also on whether a person is active or resting. A small proportion of people have blood pressures that are consistently higher than most of the community. In most cases, there is no immediate threat to health because of this, but over periods of years it is known to increase the risk of heart attacks and ruptured blood vessels in the brain (strokes). This is why it is advisable to stop the pressure from rising beyond the normal limits.

The catch is that many people's blood pressures rise when

they are in unfamiliar situations, like a doctor's surgery. There are several devices now available with which you can measure your own blood pressure easily and reliably at home. If you are worried about hypertension, buy one of these and learn to use it. Take your pressure lying in bed in the morning, when you are most relaxed, and keep a note of the readings. When you visit your doctor, take this record with you.

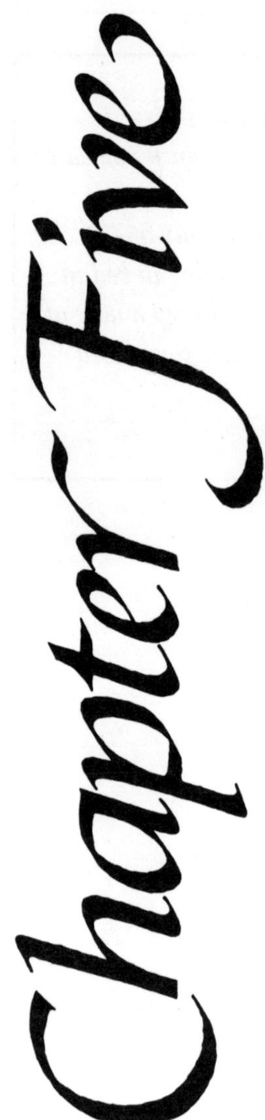

A Breath of Fresh Air

Air, like liquids, can only flow from an area of high to an area of lower pressure. So, when we breathe in, we must make the pressure inside our lungs less than it is in the atmosphere outside. Similarly, when we breathe out, the pressure inside the lung must be raised to more than atmospheric pressure.

These pressure changes are brought about by expansion or compression of the elastic bags that make up the lung. But the lung does not contain any muscle, and so it is not capable of altering size by itself. It depends entirely on the movements of the chest. Between the outside of the lung and the inside of the chest there is a slight vacuum, so that the lung is continually being sucked against the chest wall. Therefore, when the chest changes its size, the lung follows it. Breathing in, or inspiration, consists of contraction of the muscles in the diaphragm and between the ribs, which increases the volume of the chest. When these muscles relax again, the chest becomes smaller and the elastic lung shrinks back to its original size. A second set of muscles also exist, which make the chest smaller when they contract. These muscles can be used during exercise to speed up the process of breathing out.

The layer of vacuum between lung and chest, the so-called pleural space, is essential for matching lung movements to those of the chest. If the vacuum is lost by an injury to the chest wall, then the lung cannot expand during inspiratory movements, even though there may be no damage to the lung itself. This situation is called a pneumothorax. Normal function cannot be restored just by sealing up the hole in the chest: as well, a negative pressure inside the pleural cavity must be re-established by sucking out the air that has entered.

The lung is composed of small, air-filled bubbles called

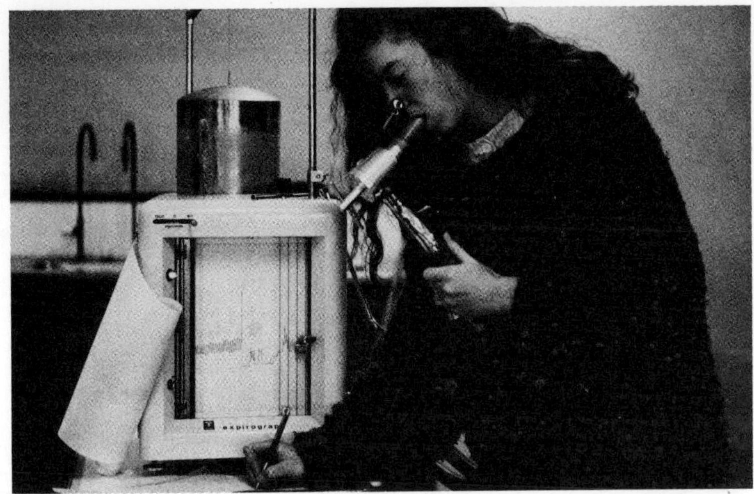

The air moving in and out of this subject's lungs can be measured if she breathes into a closed container, the volume of which is recorded on a paper chart. The apparatus is called a spirometer, and is used commonly for testing normality of lung function.

alveoli, and lung expansion involves stretching apart the components of the alveolar wall. As this happens, the alveoli become stiffer and stiffer, just as a balloon becomes progressively harder to blow up as it is inflated. The process of inspiration therefore requires quite a lot of energy.

Because respiration is a muscular action that goes on all the time, it is important to minimise the amount of energy that is needed. For this purpose, a detergent called surfactant, which reduces the stiffness of the alveoli, is released from cells in the alveolar walls every time they expand. When we are breathing only quietly, some parts of the lung are not being used, and these begin to stiffen. Yawning, which causes expansion of the whole lung, is probably a safety measure by means of which surfactant production in these areas can be stimulated.

Many victims of near-drowning, whose lungs have been filled with water, have had their stores of surfactant washed away. For about the next 24 hours, which is the period needed for the surfactant to be replaced, the lungs of these people are stiffer than normal, and they may experience difficulty in breathing. A similar problem often occurs in premature babies. Surfactant production begins only a few weeks before birth is due, so babies delivered earlier than this may have lungs that are too stiff to be expanded by their chest movements, and require artificial respiration.

Air reaches the alveoli through a branching series of tubes,

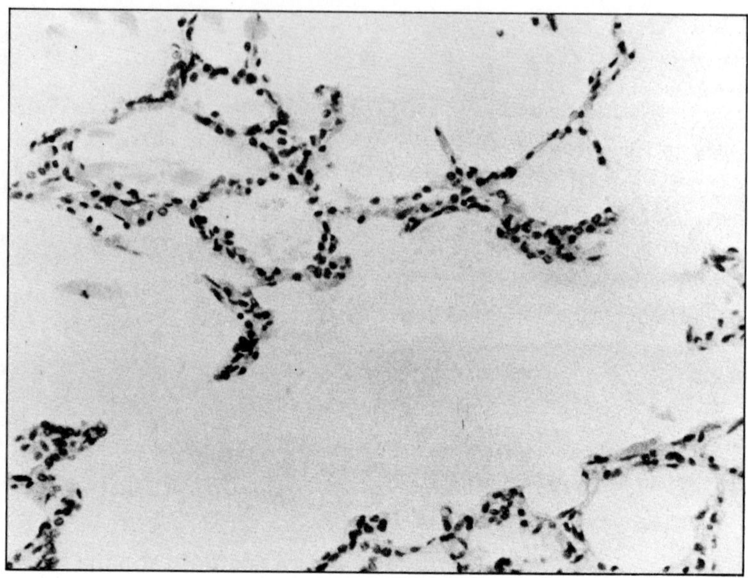

The lung is made up of millions of tiny air sacs, each with very thin walls.

consisting of the trachea or windpipe, the bronchi and the smallest branches, the bronchioles. All these tubes have a framework of cartilage, so they remain open all the time, but their walls also contain strands of muscle which can be used to alter the tube diameter and so change resistance to air flow.

The muscles of the airways are normally controlled by nerves, but they also contract in response to a variety of air-borne factors such as smoke and pollen. The difficulty in breathing that is experienced by asthmatics is because this contraction of the muscles of the airways causes a high resistance to movement of air in and out of the lung.

Sometimes another problem arises in relation to the movement of air through the airways. When we try to breathe out rapidly, for instance during exercise, the pressure created inside the lung becomes quite large, and this compresses some of the airways, so preventing efficient air movement. We may unconsciously compensate by keeping the mouth partly closed, and the lips pursed. This increases the resistance to air flow, raising the pressure in the airways and stopping them from being pressed shut by the surrounding lung.

Normally, the elastic alveolar walls help hold the airways open, like guy-ropes on a tent. If this elasticity disappears, as occurs in the lungs of many heavy smokers, then the airways collapse during even quiet expiration, with the result that breathing becomes more difficult. This condition is called emphysema.

When the lungs expand, they press on the heart and the blood vessels in the chest. As the pressure changes that normally occur during breathing are only about one-tenth of those generated by the heart, breathing does not usually have much effect on the flow of blood back into the heart from the rest of the body. But this is not always so. For instance, when somebody picks up a heavy object, the effort of lifting involves breath-holding and tensing of the thoracic muscles. The resulting pressure increase inside the chest may be great enough to completely block off the veins returning blood to the heart. When this happens, flow out of the heart also stops, and so there is no blood supply to the brain. It is therefore not surprising that people making extreme muscular efforts, such as weight lifters, sometimes faint as they try to lift an unusually heavy load.

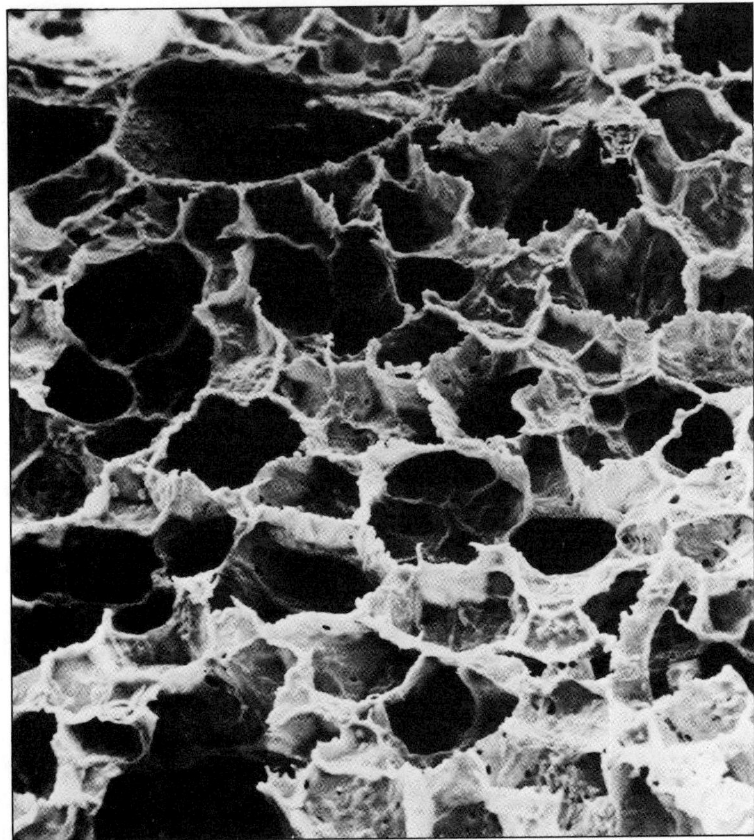

By scanning electron microscopy, we can see the structure of the lung in three dimensions. The thin-walled air sacs are connected to the outside world by a branching system of tubes. One of these is seen at the top of the picture.

The two purposes of breathing are to extract from the air the oxygen that is essential for cell metabolism, and to remove from the body carbon dioxide that is produced by these metabolic processes. Like the flow of air into the lung itself, the movements of both these gases between air, blood and cells is completely passive, depending on diffusion of gas molecules from areas of high to areas of low concentration.

Nonetheless, provision of enough oxygen to keep the body alive does require a rather special process by which the diffusion gradient can be maintained. This process involves haemoglobin, an iron-containing protein that is stored in the red blood cells. Haemoglobin has the unusual property of being able to attach to oxygen atoms very easily. Oxygen diffusing into the bloodstream from the lung is therefore continually removed from solution by binding to haemoglobin, and so the diffusion gradient for the gas from air to blood is maintained.

The haemoglobin molecules can carry about one hundred times more oxygen than could be simply dissolved in the same volume of blood. Anything that reduces the number of red blood cells or the amount of haemoglobin in them therefore endangers oxygen supply to the tissues. The poisonous gas carbon monoxide, for instance, which is contained in car exhaust fumes, binds to the oxygen-binding sites on haemoglobin much more firmly than oxygen itself does, and completely prevents oxygen carriage. Cigarette smoke also contains carbon monoxide, and the haemoglobin of heavy smokers is less able to carry oxygen than that of non-smokers.

The difficulty with using haemoglobin to carry most of the oxygen from lungs to organs is persuading it to let go again, as the oxygen-haemoglobin complex is a very stable one. Fortunately, this stability is weakened in acid conditions, and the environment of cells is always acidic, because of the nature of most cell waste products. The acid diffuses into the nearby blood vessels, splitting the oxygen-haemoglobin complex, and allowing the free oxygen to diffuse out of the blood stream to the cells.

In pregnancy, the circulations of baby and mother are separate, and oxygen transfer to the baby's blood stream involves yet another diffusion process. This slows down access of oxygen to

A radiographic section through the heart shows the coronary arteries spreading between the heart muscle cells. Blockage of any of these coronary branches will deprive an area of muscle of its oxygen supply, and cause a heart attack.

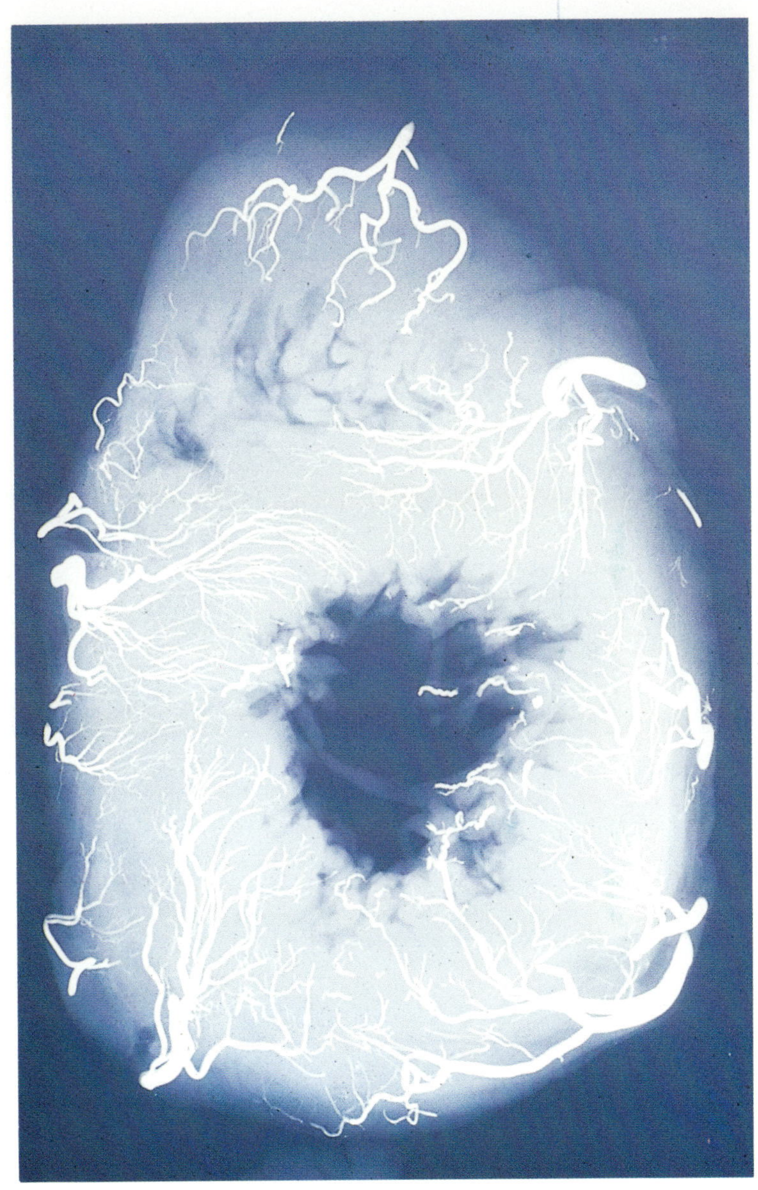

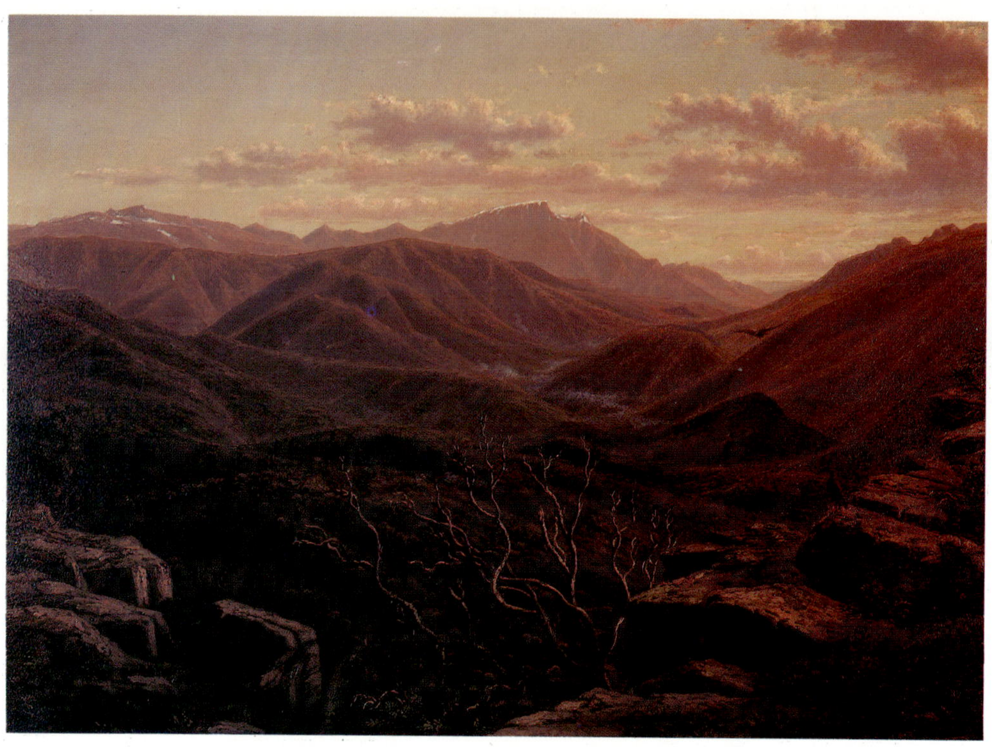

As one ascends from sea level to higher altitudes, the amount of oxygen available in the air decreases. People who live at high altitudes show important adaptive changes in order to cope with this problem. No mountains in Australia, however, are high enough for these changes to occur. Eagle's View of the Mountains: Head of the Mitta Mitta, *E. von Guerard. La Trobe Library.*

The abdominal cavity is almost entirely filled by the intestines and liver, as shown in this intricate life-size model made in Germany around 1900. All the individual organs are removable. The liver is the reddish organ at the top of the abdominal cavity, and the green gall bladder can be seen just below it.

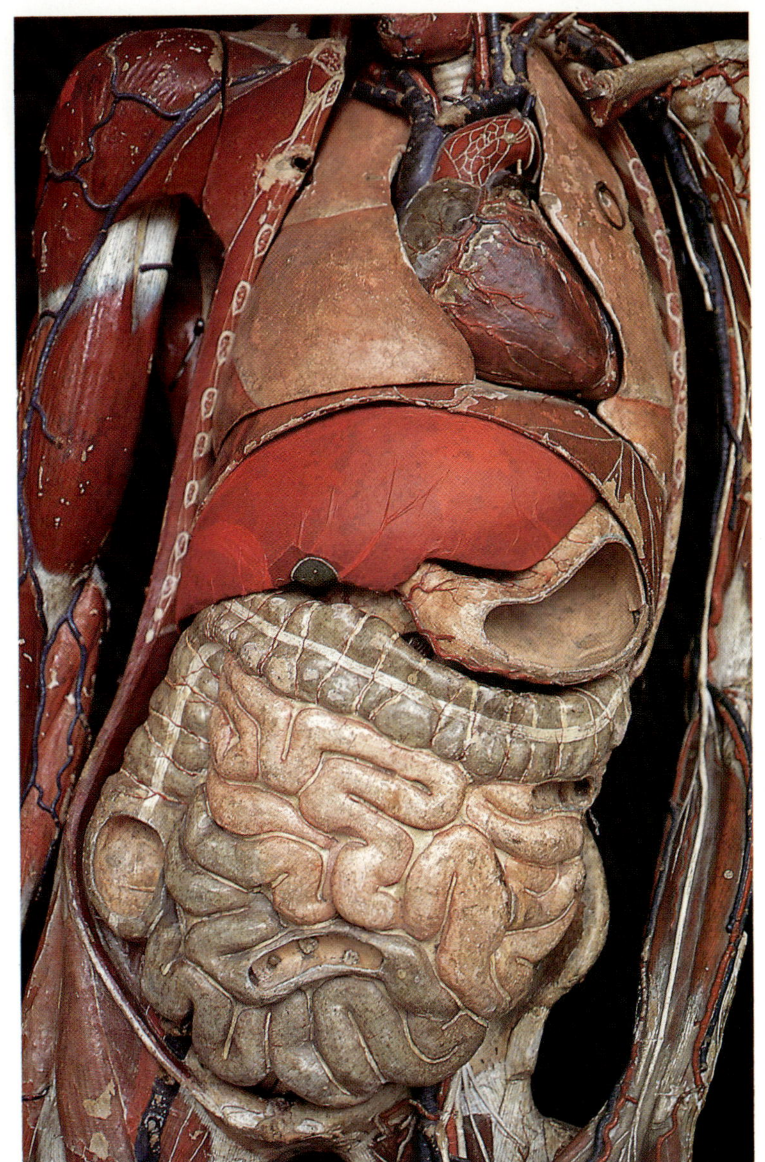

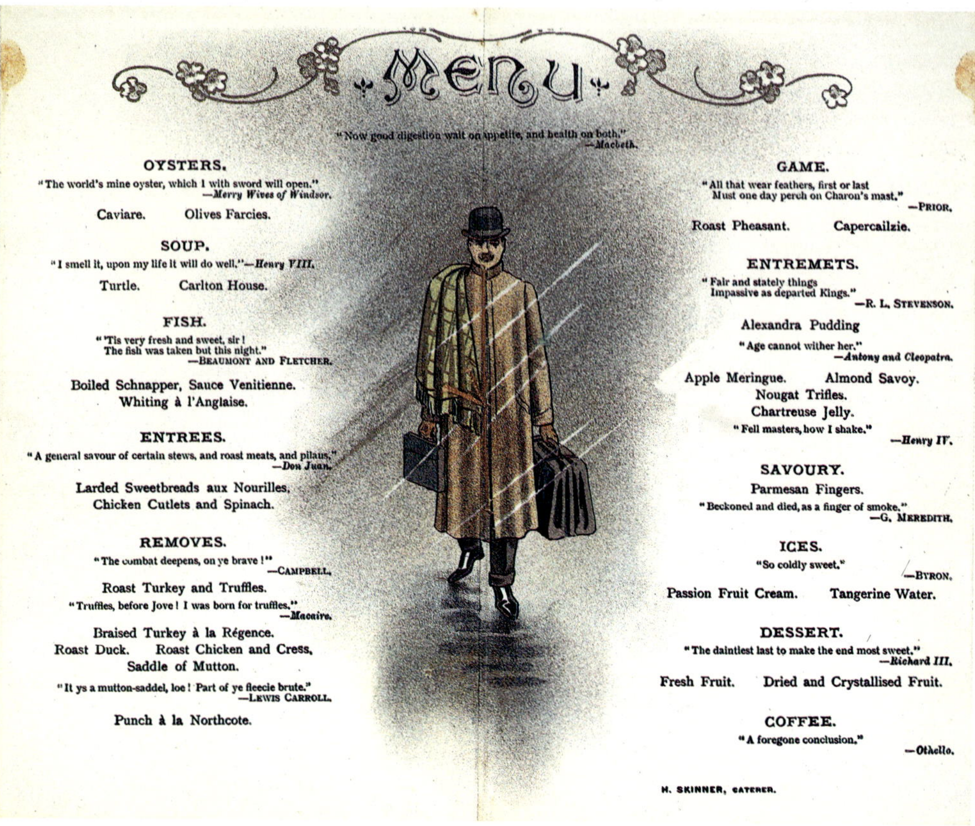

MENU

"Now good digestion wait on appetite, and health on both."
—Macbeth.

OYSTERS.

"The world's mine oyster, which I with sword will open."
—*Merry Wives of Windsor.*

Caviare. Olives Farcies.

SOUP.

"I smell it, upon my life it will do well."—*Henry VIII.*

Turtle. Carlton House.

FISH.

"'Tis very fresh and sweet, sir!
The fish was taken but this night."
—BEAUMONT AND FLETCHER.

Boiled Schnapper, Sauce Venitienne.
Whiting à l'Anglaise.

ENTREES.

"A general savour of certain stews, and roast meats, and pilaus."
—*Don Juan.*

Larded Sweetbreads aux Nourilles.
Chicken Cutlets and Spinach.

REMOVES.

"The combat deepens, on ye brave!"
—CAMPBELL.

Roast Turkey and Truffles.

"Truffles, before Jove! I was born for truffles."
—*Macaire.*

Braised Turkey à la Régence.
Roast Duck. Roast Chicken and Cress.
Saddle of Mutton.

"It ys a mutton-saddel, loe! Part of ye fleecie brute."
—LEWIS CARROLL.

Punch à la Northcote.

GAME.

"All that wear feathers, first or last
Must one day perch on Charon's mast."
—PRIOR.

Roast Pheasant. Capercailzie.

ENTREMETS.

"Fair and stately things
Impassive as departed Kings."
—R. L. STEVENSON.

Alexandra Pudding

"Age cannot wither her."
—*Antony and Cleopatra.*

Apple Meringue. Almond Savoy.
Nougat Trifles.
Chartreuse Jelly.

"Fell masters, how I shake."
—*Henry IV.*

SAVOURY.

Parmesan Fingers.

"Beckoned and died, as a finger of smoke."
—G. MEREDITH.

ICES.

"So coldly sweet."
—BYRON.

Passion Fruit Cream. Tangerine Water.

DESSERT.

"The daintiest last to make the end most sweet."
—*Richard III.*

Fresh Fruit. Dried and Crystallised Fruit.

COFFEE.

"A foregone conclusion."
—*Othello.*

H. SKINNER, CATERER.

The nutritional value of food is independent of how it tastes, but our appetite for food depends to a large extent on its taste and its appearance, as well as on the formalities that accompany a meal. Commercial Traveller's Association menu. *La Trobe Library.*

the foetal bloodstream. The baby compensates by making haemoglobin molecules that are slightly different from the adult protein, and are able to bind oxygen better. Over the twelve months after birth, the molecular structure changes gradually to the adult form. During this period, therefore, the proportions of each haemoglobin provides an index of a baby's age. One of the central controversies in the recent Chamberlain murder case revolved around the accuracy of tests used to distinguish the two types.

Oxygen always constitutes twenty-one per cent of atmospheric air, regardless of altitude. However, with increasing height above sea level the concentrations of all gases present become less and less, so the total amount of available oxygen falls. People who live at high altitudes show dramatic compensatory responses to this. Their blood contains about thirty per cent more red blood cells than normal, and they have enlarged lungs and chests, so they can take much deeper breaths. Above a certain altitude, however, even these compensations cannot provide enough oxygen to keep the body's cells alive. Interestingly enough, this critical altitude corresponds almost exactly to the highest point on Earth, Mount Everest.

People who live at sea level and ascend to high altitudes suffer attacks of nausea, vomiting and dizziness, known as mountain sickness, for several days after their arrival. These non-acclimatised individuals undoubtedly have an oxygen deficiency, but breathing oxygen or returning to low altitude does not produce an immediate cure. So the unpleasant symptoms are not due directly to lack of oxygen. Instead, mountain sickness seems to be due mainly to the reduced barometric pressure, which no longer compresses the blood vessels of the brain as much as occurs at low altitude. This allows fluid to leak from the blood into the brain, with subsequent effects on neighbouring nerve cells. Fortunately, mountain sickness never occurs in Australia. The minimum altitude that produces the illness is about 3000 metres, while our highest mountain, Mount Kosciusko, is just over 2000 metres high.

An excess of oxygen can be just as dangerous as its absence. The body's cells are designed to function best at oxygen concentrations like those normally in the atmosphere. When this concentration is raised, then some parts of the cellular machinery are oxidised and stop working, in the same way as metals oxidise, or rust, when exposed to oxygen in the air.

But under some circumstances, the danger of breathing pure oxygen has to be balanced against its benefits. For instance, some premature babies are just not able to absorb enough oxygen from normal air, because of their immature lungs. To survive, therefore, they have to be kept for a time in an oxygen-enriched environment. Again, where self-contained breathing supplies are needed, in space craft for example, pure oxygen is obviously less bulky to carry than air. The astronauts on the Apollo missions breathed pure oxygen, but at a pressure only about one-third that at sea level, which reduced its toxicity and also the danger of an explosion. The more recent Space Shuttles, by contrast, have routinely carried supplies of normal air, at normal atmospheric pressure.

The process of breathing is controlled by the nervous system, and the nerve cells that are involved lie in an area of the base of the brain called the pons, at about the level of the ear lobes. These neurons (nerve cells) are divided into two groups, and the cells of each group fire bursts of electrical activity every few seconds, but out of phase with each other. The first group sends instructions to the muscles responsible for inspiration, and the time taken to breathe in corresponds to the period for which these neurons are active. At the end of inspiration, the second group of cells starts to fire. These neurons switch off the contractions of the inspiratory muscles, allowing the chest to relax and producing expiration. With deep breathing, for instance in exercise, the expiratory neurons not only terminate inspiration but as well cause contraction of a second set of muscles, which speeds the movement of air out of the lung.

As the role of breathing is to carry oxygen and carbon dioxide around the body, it is not surprising that the pattern of respiratory neuron activity is affected by the concentrations of these gases dissolved in the blood. Either decreasing the blood oxygen or increasing the blood carbon dioxide will increase firing of the inspiratory neurons, and so increase the volume of air breathed, until the blood gas levels are restored to normal.

Because oxygen is essential to life, we might expect that a lack of this gas would be the main stimulus to breathing. However, haemoglobin is so efficient at carrying oxygen that quite large changes in dissolved blood oxygen have only small effects on tissue function. So it is unnecessary to maintain the dissolved oxygen concentration at a constant value, and the brain only detects dramatic falls. By contrast, very slight changes in blood carbon dioxide affect tissue function profoundly. Carbon dioxide concentration alters the acidity, or pH, of the tissue fluids, and variations in pH result in dramatic changes to many biochemical processes. It is therefore essential that the carbon dioxide levels in the blood are closely controlled.

The relative importance of the two gases in stimulating respiration can be seen by measuring the time for which one can hold one's breath under different circumstances. Normally, breath-holding time depends on how long it takes for the blood carbon dioxide to build up to a level that stimulates the inspiratory neurons. If one over-breathes, or hyperventilates, for about ten breaths, almost all of the carbon dioxide in the blood is blown off into the air. Now inspiration will not be initiated until the blood oxygen falls to the low level necessary to cause brain stimulation, so it is possible to hold one's breath for perhaps three or four times as long as before.

Snorkel divers routinely use this trick to prolong their diving time, but it can be hazardous: if all the blood carbon dioxide is blown off, then the blood oxygen level may fall so far before it triggers any urge to breathe that the diver loses consciousness.

While the total amount of air entering and leaving the lung is controlled by the dissolved gases in the bloodstream, ventilation of particular areas of the lung is regulated by local gas concentrations in the small airways. When one is breathing quietly, not all the alveoli are being ventilated, with the result that in the stagnant area the concentration of carbon dioxide rises, and that of oxygen falls. These changes in gas concentration relax the muscles in the airway walls, with a fall of airway resistance. At the same time, nerves in the airways detect the abnormal gas mixture and stimulate the yawning reflex. The combination of reduced airway resistance and increased air intake produces better ventilation of the stagnant region, so local gas levels are restored to normal.

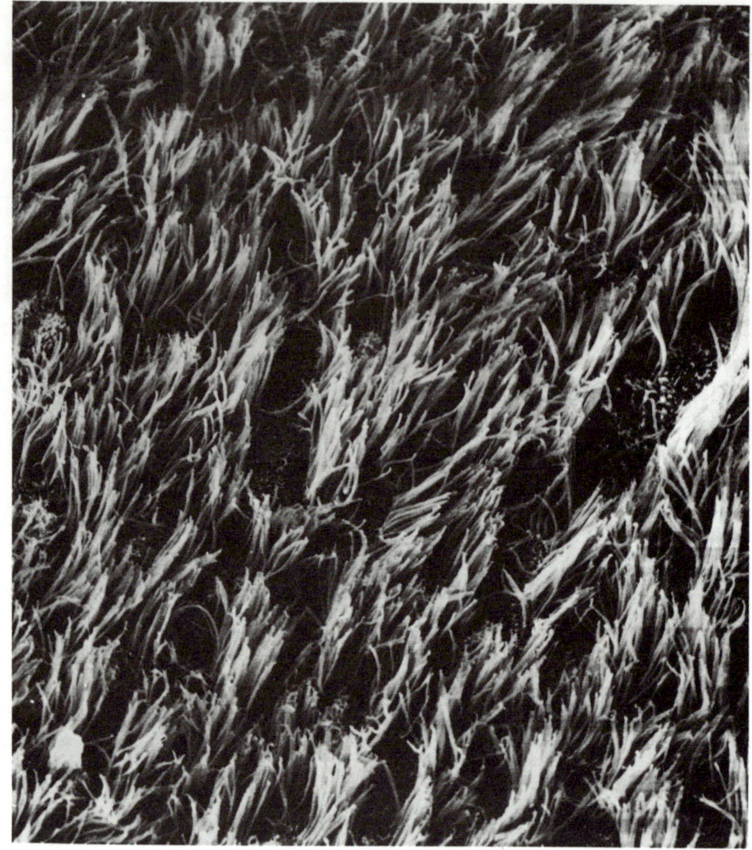

The airways that carry air in and out of the lung are lined with tiny hairs, or cilia. Continual movements of these cilia are essential for clearing mucous secretions and inhaled particles out of the airways, so they do not block up the air sacs and prevent gas exchange.

During sleep, there may be even more dramatic changes in breathing patterns. Quite often, relaxation of the muscles of the mouth and throat causes them to collapse over the trachea and obstruct air movement. As air is sucked past the obstruction, vibrations are set up, producing the sound we know as snoring. In some people, there is so much obstruction to air flow that large amounts of carbon dioxide build up in the bloodstream. These individuals characteristically have periods of sleep during which they snore very loudly, separated by brief periods when so much carbon dioxide has accumulated that they wake up and take a deep breath.

The tragedy of cot death may reflect a deficiency in this safety mechanism. It has been suggested that in babies the brain pathways that produce waking in response to elevated blood carbon dioxide may not yet be fully developed. So while an older child would wake up if an obstruction to breathing caused a dangerous build up of carbon dioxide, a baby might not.

Recently, a Yugoslavian scientist, Franco Kajfez, has developed a herbal medicine that is claimed to stop snoring. A snore is almost always linked to breathing through the mouth rather than the nose. Kajfez thinks that mouth-breathing during sleep occurs only when the mucous membranes in the nose become dried out, and his potion is designed to keep these membranes moist. Whether the theory is right or not, international drug companies are rumoured to be very interested.

Apart from snoring, the most familiar normal change in breathing is probably the hyperventilation associated with exercise. When we exercise, the volume of air moved in and out of the lungs rises in proportion to the amount of work being done. The amount of energy used to drive the respiratory muscles also rises, from an insignificant value at rest to about twenty per cent of our total energy expenditure during maximal exertion. Despite this, the ability for gas exchange in the lung is normally never a limiting factor in exercise. Rather, exercise capacity is governed by how much blood can be pumped by the heart, or in other words how quickly the gases can be transported around the body.

The mechanism by which respiration increases in proportion to physical work load has been a controversial subject for many years. The blood gas concentrations during exercise are similar to those at rest, and anyway breathing increases at the beginning of exercise, before any change in blood gases could occur. So the hyperventilation cannot be primarily a response to increased oxygen usage or to increased carbon dioxide excretion by the working muscles.

In a resting person, passive movement of the limbs stimulates breathing, suggesting that detection of exercise by the brian might underlie the initial response as movement commences. But the size of this effect is not enough to explain the ten to fifteen-fold increase in gas exchange that occurs during sustained exercise. Here, it is possible that the brain centres which control muscle movement and body temperature interact with the neurons that control respiration. However, the complete answer still evades us.

THE SINISTER SNORE

At up to seventy decibels, the human snore is about as loud as a road drill. But as well as being irritating to other people, snorers may be a danger to themselves.

Because it is caused by tissues collapsing over the trachea and obstructing it, and the necks of fat people contain more soft tissue, snoring is often a symptom of being overweight. The heavy snorer may also intermittently develop complete obstruction of the respiratory passages, waking up and taking a breath only when blood carbon dioxide levels rise enough to stimulate the brain.

As we have to be awake for about fifteen seconds before we remember it next morning, the sufferer from this so-called 'sleep apnoea' is unlikely to know that sleep was continually being interrupted, but will still be tired during the day and so may be prone to accidents. As well, sleep apnoea is known to be associated with high blood pressure: about thirty per cent of hypertensive patients have the syndrome. Whether the respiratory disturbance helps to cause high blood pressure, or whether the two phenomena are just linked to another factor such as obesity, is still not known. Nevertheless, the evidence suggests that snoring is a health hazard.

THE CHALLENGE OF BREATHING UNDERWATER

Along with the lure of being able to fly, mankind's greatest obsession has been survival beneath the sea.

Self-contained underwater breathing apparatus (SCUBA) is widely used both by professional and sporting divers. With this system, normal room air is breathed from a back-pack. But the pressures encountered underwater are very high because of the high density of water: every ten metre change in depth corresponds to a change in altitude on land of about twenty kilometres! These enormous pressures exerted on the gas contained within the lungs, bloodstream and body tissues of a diver make the situation quite different to that experienced above water.

The most serious problem involves a gas that makes up eighty per cent of normal room air, but is often ignored because it is not used or produced by the body. This gas is nitrogen. Nitrogen is not as soluble in water as are oxygen or carbon dioxide, but when the body is pressurised by the weight of surrounding water, then large quantities of nitrogen dissolve in the tissues, just as the bubbles in champagne are dissolved so long as the bottle is sealed. Rapid ascent to the surface will then be similar to opening the champagne bottle: nitrogen comes out of solution and forms bubbles. If these are large enough, they can block blood vessels, producing pain and damage in the tissues deprived of blood. To prevent this occurring, it is important that SCUBA divers ascend towards the surface in stages. This allows time for accumulated tissue nitrogen to diffuse into the lungs without forming large bubbles. The amount of

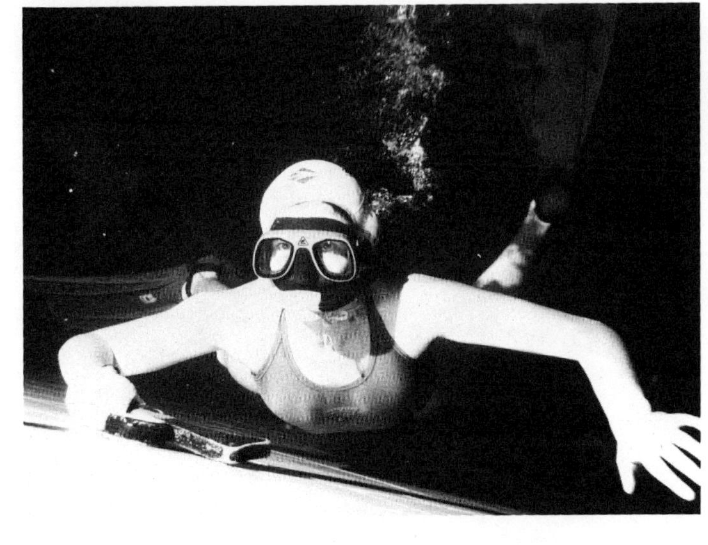

Man has always been fascinated by the challenge of breathing underwater. Mastering the ability to extract oxygen from the water instead of having to carry it in gas form would be a great advance in treating the breathing problems of premature babies, as well as being useful to this underwater hockey player.

time needed for this decompression after deep dives may be much longer than the dive itself. For instance, after ninety minutes spent at a depth of sixty metres, a total of five hours must be spent travelling back to the surface.

The dangers of breathing gas at high pressure have led to attempts to substitute an inert liquid as the vehicle for carrying oxygen into the lungs. Animals immersed in liquid fluorocarbon saturated with oxygen have survived, and been able to return to air-breathing afterwards. Although the technique has not yet been perfected for human use, it would be of great help in the treatment of premature babies, who lack lung surfactant. Removal of the gas-liquid interface within the alveoli would abolish the high surface tension that usually prevents the lungs of these babies expanding when they breathe.

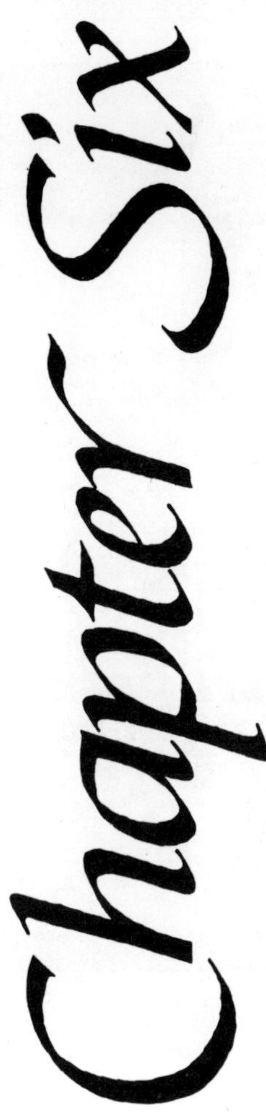

Stoking Up the Furnace

To understand the organ systems in our bodies it is often helpful to think about them in terms of machinery, as well as collections of living cells. Although, of course, this is a great oversimplification, it emphasises the underlying purposes of the systems.

The digestive tract, for example, is really rather like a chemical extraction plant such as is used for purifying gold ore, although it is concerned with separation of different organic molecules rather than with separation of minerals.

To start the process, the material to be processed is crushed and ground to a slurry in a mill of some sort – in this case the mouth. It then runs into a settling tank, the stomach, where some preliminary sorting out and chemical treatment occurs so as to get rid of the most easily separated rubbish. This process involves exposure of the food to enzymes and acid, which begin to break down the particles into their constituent molecules, and kill any bacteria that are present.

Next, the prepared material passes on to the extraction plant of the intestine, where applications of more chemicals release the substances of value so they can be removed and purified. As food moves down the intestine, powerful digestive enzymes are secreted into it, and rhythmic contractions of the intestinal wall stir the mixture around. Nutrients that have been released by enzyme action are then absorbed into the bloodstream by specialised transport systems in the wall.

Finally, we need to get rid of any waste material left over from the extraction process. In the case of gold ore, unfortunately for the mining companies, very little precious metal is found in proportion to the amount of waste that has to be dumped on the mullock heap. By contrast, our digestive extraction processes produce a very high yield of nutrients. While we eat perhaps a

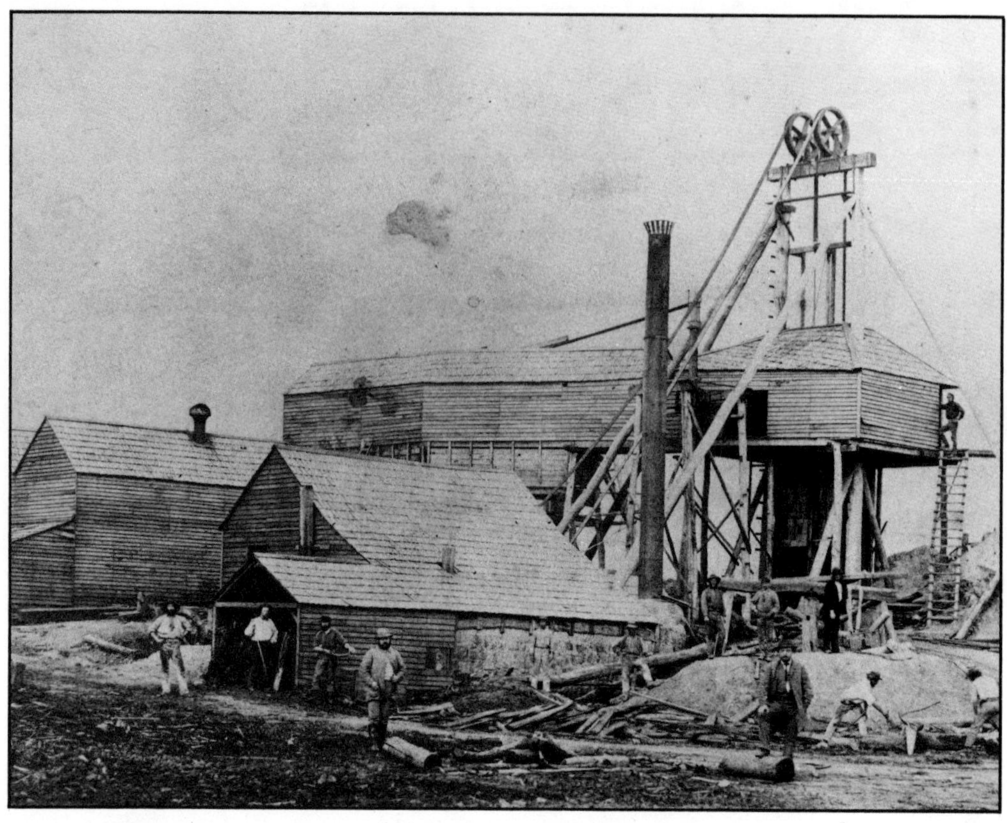

During the 1860s, mines like this one in the Victorian countryside between Ballarat and Bendigo extracted thousands of ounces of gold from the underlying rock. The sequence of processes used to extract gold from base rock are rather similar to those which occur in the stomach and intestines after a meal. Brown's & Smythe's Mining Co., Smythesdale, *c. 1861, Solomon & Bardwell. La Trobe Library.*

kilogram of food per day, only about fifty grams of this is passed as faeces. The remaining ninety-five per cent has been absorbed.

Not only nutrients are absorbed as food passes down the intestine. Our daily intake of fluid is about two litres, and the digestive glands pour substantially larger amounts into various parts of the digestive tract over the same period. For instance, continual salivary secretion is necessary to keep the mouth lubricated so that we can speak. Saliva is also needed to help us swallow food. Daily secretion from these glands is about one and a half litres. A further four or more litres of watery secretions enter the stomach and intestine during the day, making a total of over seven litres. But the faeces contain only about one-tenth of a litre of water: almost all of this seven litres has therefore been reabsorbed again.

The reabsorption of water takes place in the lower part of the intestine, the colon. The longer the time waste material lies in this region, the more reabsorption will occur. Normally, waves of contraction, or peristalsis, regularly travel along the intestine and move the wastes from a particular meal out of the colon over one or two days. These peristaltic movements are initiated by the intestinal contents stretching the colon wall.

Sometimes, when the bulk of material present is not enough to stretch the colon sufficiently, peristalsis does not occur, so the wastes lie in the colon for longer than usual and more water is removed. The result is that the faeces become dried out and constipation results. The most effective way of preventing constipation is to eat a diet that is high in fibre. Because the digestive enzymes cannot break down fibre, a greater bulk of material enters the colon, ensuring that the wall is stretched enough for peristaltic movements to be set off.

Under some other circumstances, less water than normal is reabsorbed. For instance, certain bacteria that produce food poisoning, such as *E. Coli*, *Salmonella* and 'golden staph', produce toxins that block the water reabsorbing pumps. This not only

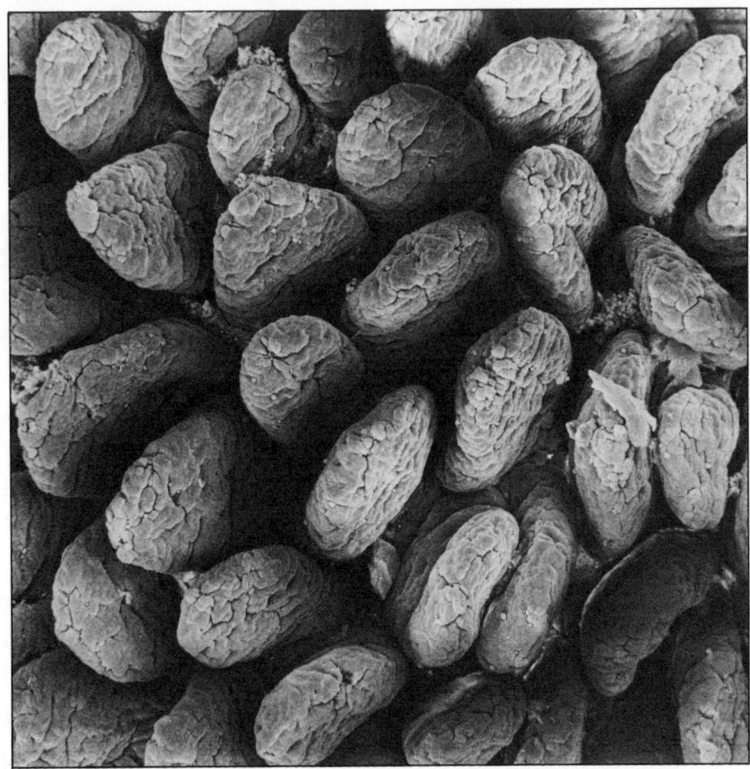

To maximise the efficiency with which food is absorbed, the lining of the intestine is covered with tiny finger-like projections, providing a very large total surface area. Each projection is rich in blood capillaries and possesses specialised pumps for transporting food molecules.

prevents the normal solidification of the faeces, but also stimulates peristalsis because of the increased volume of material present. The result is diarrhoea. The profound diarrhoea caused by cholera bacteria kills at least ten million children in the Third World every year, simply due to the dehydration resulting from intestinal water loss. But also, if it goes on long enough, less extreme diarrhoea can produce serious dehydration too. As well, food is moved through the intestine too fast for normal absorption, so malnutrition may result as the body's stores of energy-giving fuels run down.

Although many parts of the body behave as factories for the production of specific substances, there is one organ that stands out as the most complex and hard-working factory of all – the liver.

The liver not only works harder than most other organs, but it is bigger as well; at about 1·5 kilograms, it is the largest single organ in the body. It has many different functions that make it essential for life, all of which are related to the peculiar organisation of its blood supply. For while every other organ is nourished by blood coming in arteries from the heart and lungs, most of the blood supply for the liver comes through the veins that are returning blood from the digestive tract. So everything that is absorbed from the intestine during digestion must pass through the liver before it reaches the rest of the body.

This unique anatomical arrangement makes the liver an ideal guard post for detecting any poisonous substances that may have been eaten. The cells that line the blood vessels inside the liver contain enzymes that destroy many different sorts of molecules, and help to purify the blood as it passes through. Alcohol is one of the molecules that is destroyed to a large extent within the liver. So when the liver is damaged by infection, for instance in hepatitis, drinking even small amounts of alcohol may produce serious intoxication.

The enzymes that inactivate ingested poisons have other purposes as well. For instance, they attack some vitamins that are absorbed from the intestine in a biologically inactive form, changing them to molecules that are usable by the body.

A second function of the liver is to make proteins for release into the bloodstream. Some of these proteins are essential for the process of blood clotting; others have the basic role of attracting water molecules around them, and so keep the volume of blood constant. If the amount of protein in the bloodstream falls, then water leaks out of the blood vessels into the spaces between the body's cells, and into the abdomen, causing the swelling known as oedema. Oedema will also result if the diet does not contain enough of the amino acids that are necessary for protein synthesis: children suffering from starvation often have distended bellies, because of the water that has leaked out of their blood.

Storage of valuable nutrients is another of the liver's roles. Almost all the body's chemical processes use the simple carbohydrate, glucose, as fuel, and enough glucose is stored here to keep the body running for about three hours. Large quantities of some vitamins are also stored in the liver. For instance, it contains enough vitamin B_{12} to last the body for four years! These enormous amounts of vitamins are one of the reasons why liver is such a nutritious foodstuff.

Finally, absorption of some important foodstuffs across the wall of the intestine itself depends on the liver. The fats in our food, being insoluble in water, stick onto the intestinal lining just as grease clings to plates when you wash up without enough detergent. The body's detergent is bile, which is made in the liver and released into the intestine through the gall bladder and bile duct. There it dissolves the fats that have been eaten and allows them to be taken into the bloodstream.

Bile is greenish-brown in colour, because of the presence of pigments originating from breakdown of the haemoglobin in dying blood cells. The same pigments produce the characteristic colours of our urine and faeces. Because blood cells have only a short life span, haemoglobin breakdown is occurring all the time, and the pigments are continually filtered out of the bloodstream by the liver. If, however, the blood cells are destroyed more rapidly by infection, or if the liver is damaged, then the blood takes on the colour of the pigments, and the person begins to look yellowish, or 'jaundiced'.

The normal liver contains many more cells than are needed for its various functions, which is all to the good considering that it has to purify everything we eat and drink. As well, it is able to grow new cells when damage occurs. However, these are often not able to function effectively, as they have no access to the bloodstream. A large liver is therefore not necessarily a useful one. This is dramatically illustrated in alcoholic cirrhosis, where the liver is often greatly swollen, but has very little capacity to perform its normal jobs. So, severe alcoholism is often associated with loss of blood proteins, with vitamin deficiency and with malnutrition due to lack of absorption of fats.

In order to obtain energy from foodstuffs, the food molecules must be reacted with oxygen (oxidation). This is really identical to burning the same substances in an environment containing oxygen, such as air. So measuring how much heat is produced by burning a food tells us how much energy the body could obtain from it.

In the same way we can determine how much energy a person is using up. One method of doing this is to measure how much heat the person produces, but this is accurate only under some circumstances, and requires an expensive insulated room in which to put the person. A simpler way is to measure the rate at which oxygen is used for the oxidation process. As we know the concentration of oxygen in room air, we only need to collect in a bag the air that the person breathes out, and measure how much lower the oxygen content is. Typically, a resting person uses up all the oxygen from about one litre of air every minute.

Energy expenditure, or how fast our metabolic processes are working, is called the metabolic rate, and in a resting person this is about equivalent to the energy used by a 75 Watt light bulb. When we exercise, however, we may need up to twenty times more energy than this, and therefore we need to increase the amount of metabolic fuel that is available.

As most chemical processes in the body use glucose as fuel, it is important that the amount of this sugar circulating through the bloodstream is kept fairly constant, even though food intake may occur only two or three times a day.

One safety mechanism that has evolved is the ability to store the glucose that has been absorbed from the diet but is not needed for immediate energy. Some storage occurs in the liver and the muscles, but most is in the fatty tissues of the body. So, in cold climates, fat serves a double purpose; insulating the body and providing a source of metabolic heat.

Release of the hormone insulin from the pancreas is a second safety mechanism helping to ensure a regular supply of glucose. Insulin stops glucose being freed from its stores in the body, and so reduces the amount circulating in the bloodstream. The trigger for insulin release is a rise in blood glucose, such as after a meal. When this extra glucose has been used up, and the amount in the bloodstream start to fall again, insulin release is turned off and more glucose can be freed from storage areas.

Without insulin, there is no way of providing a steady supply of glucose to the body, and death results. The vital role of insulin was discovered by a group of Canadian scientists in 1921, when they showed that a dog without a pancreas could be kept healthy if it was injected with pancreas extract. Soon after, the same extract was able to be tested in diabetic patients and was shown to be life-saving. Since that time, insulin has probably saved more animal and human lives than any other medicine except penicillin.

Despite their efficiency, the mechanisms that regulate glucose in the bloodstream can function only if the body's stores of glucose and other nutrients are replenished. So the factors that control food intake are also a necessary part of our metabolism.

The basis of food appetite is complex, because it includes psychological as well as physiological influences. We all know that preferences for particular foods, and the appearance and smell of a meal, have very powerful effects on how much we eat. But there must also be some way of detecting whether the body needs nutrients. Once again, glucose probably plays an important part in this, with rises of blood glucose after eating causing a loss of appetite.

Over periods of months or years, additional factors may influence food intake, because most people show remarkably constant body weights even though their food intake and energy expenditure may vary enormously from time to time. There is evidence that individuals adjust their food intake so as to keep their total body fat stores at a particular level, which is high for some people and low for others. This might explain why maintained weight reduction is for most people very difficult to achieve. It also suggests one important cause of obesity. When we are adult, overfeeding increases the storage of fat in the existing cells of our adipose tissues, but does not change the number of these cells. In children, by contrast, excess food intake causes the fat cells to multiply. So a man who is overfed as a child will have a permanently increased capacity for fat storage, and is likely to regulate his body weight accordingly.

DAILY REQUIREMENTS FOR ESSENTIAL VITAMINS

This is a list of the main foods containing high levels of the vitamins that are essential to health, and an indication of what quantity of various foodstuffs contain the daily quota of these substances. However, even if you don't eat the particular foods listed here, most balanced diets still provide enough vitamins for a healthy adult. Growing children and woman who are pregnant or breast-feeding, on the other hand, may need to pay greater attention to how adequate their intakes are.

Vitamin	Main sources	Sample daily requirement
A	*animal fats, liver, dairy products, carrots*	*150 g cheddar cheese OR 50 g liver OR 10 g carrot*
B group		
B_1	*yeast, cereal germ, pulses*	*50 g wheat germ OR 200 g rolled oats OR 100 g dried peas OR 1 teaspoon Vegemite*

riboflavine	*liver, beef, lamb, pork, eggs*	*50g liver OR 150g kidney OR 1 teaspoon Vegemite*
folic acid	*dark green vegetables, liver, kidney*	*150g liver OR 200g kidney OR 200g spinach or 1 teaspoon Vegemite*
B_{12}	*all meats, milk*	*200g lean beef OR 2 eggs*
nicotinic acid	*meat organs, fish, whole cereals, pulses*	*300g lean beef OR 100g liver OR 200g oily fish OR 100g peanuts*
C	*citrus fruit, berries, some brassicas*	*150ml fresh orange juice OR 100g strawberries OR 100g broccoli*
D	*animal fats*	*50g oily fish (salmon, herring) OR 1 egg*

(Data adapted from Scientific Tables, 8th edition, Ciba-Geigy, 1981.)

DESIRABLE BODY WEIGHTS

The weights of adults vary widely, depending partly on body build, partly on lifestyle and partly on other factors. The question of whether one is 'overweight' is therefore often a matter of interpretation. Life insurance statistics suggest that the figures given overpage are 'desirable' weight ranges for males and females of different heights (wearing indoor clothing, with shoes). If you are more than ten per cent heavier than the maximum weight suggested for your height, you should seriously consider a weight reduction programme in order to remain in good health. To convert pounds to kilograms, halve your weight in pounds and subtract ten per cent.

Women

Height		*Weight (kg)*	
(cm)	*Small frame*	*Medium frame*	*Large frame*
150	*43–46*	*46–51*	*48–55*
155	*45–49*	*47–53*	*51–58*
160	*47–51*	*50–55*	*54–61*
165	*50–54*	*49–59*	*49–64*
170	*54–58*	*56–63*	*60–68*
175	*57–61*	*60–67*	*64–72*
180	*61–65*	*64–70*	*68–76*

Men

Height		*Weight (kg)*	
(cm)	*Small frame*	*Medium frame*	*Large frame*
160	*52–56*	*55–60*	*59–65*
165	*55–59*	*57–63*	*61–69*
170	*58–62*	*61–67*	*64–73*
175	*62–66*	*64–71*	*69–77*
180	*65–70*	*68–75*	*72–81*
185	*69–74*	*72–79*	*76–86*
190	*73–78*	*75–84*	*81–90*

(Data from the Statistical Bulletin of the Metropolitan Life Insurance Office.)

Chapter Seven

The Quintessential Filter

Cooks have a good idea of the structure of the human kidney, because, cut in half, it looks very similar to the sheep's kidney. The outer part is dark, and pinkish in colour. This dark tissue consists of tiny tubes, or tubules, called nephrons. One end of each tubule wraps around a spherical cluster of blood capillaries, forming a structure called a glomerulus. The glomerulus filters water and dissolved substances out of the bloodstream into the tubule, where they are processed into urine.

The other end of each tubule drains urine into the pale area in the centre of the kidney. Here the urine is collected, and then runs through the ureter to the bladder. There are about a million nephrons in one kidney, each one about six centimetres long. So the two kidneys of a healthy person contain about 120 kilometres, or 75 miles, of tubules.

Fluid moves from the bloodstream into the tubules because of the high concentrations of dissolved substances like sodium chloride (salt) in the blood. The particles of salt diffuse rapidly into the tubular fluid and pull large numbers of water molecules along with them. Every day, about 200 litres of water and a kilogram of salt pass out of the bloodstream in this way.

Other substances can also diffuse across into the tubules. In diabetes, the blood contains a high concentration of glucose. So here both water and glucose are lost into the urine, and a diabetic person therefore often suffers from severe thirst and dehydration.

As well, the amount of fluid that is filtered depends on how much blood is flowing through the glomerular capillaries. Most people notice that urine production is greater in cold weather; this is because cold shuts off the blood vessels to the skin, allowing more blood to flow through other parts of the body, including the kidneys.

Nature has devised safety measures to ensure that vital organs in our bodies can maintain their function. In the case of the kidneys, duplication provides a large safety margin for adequate control of blood composition.

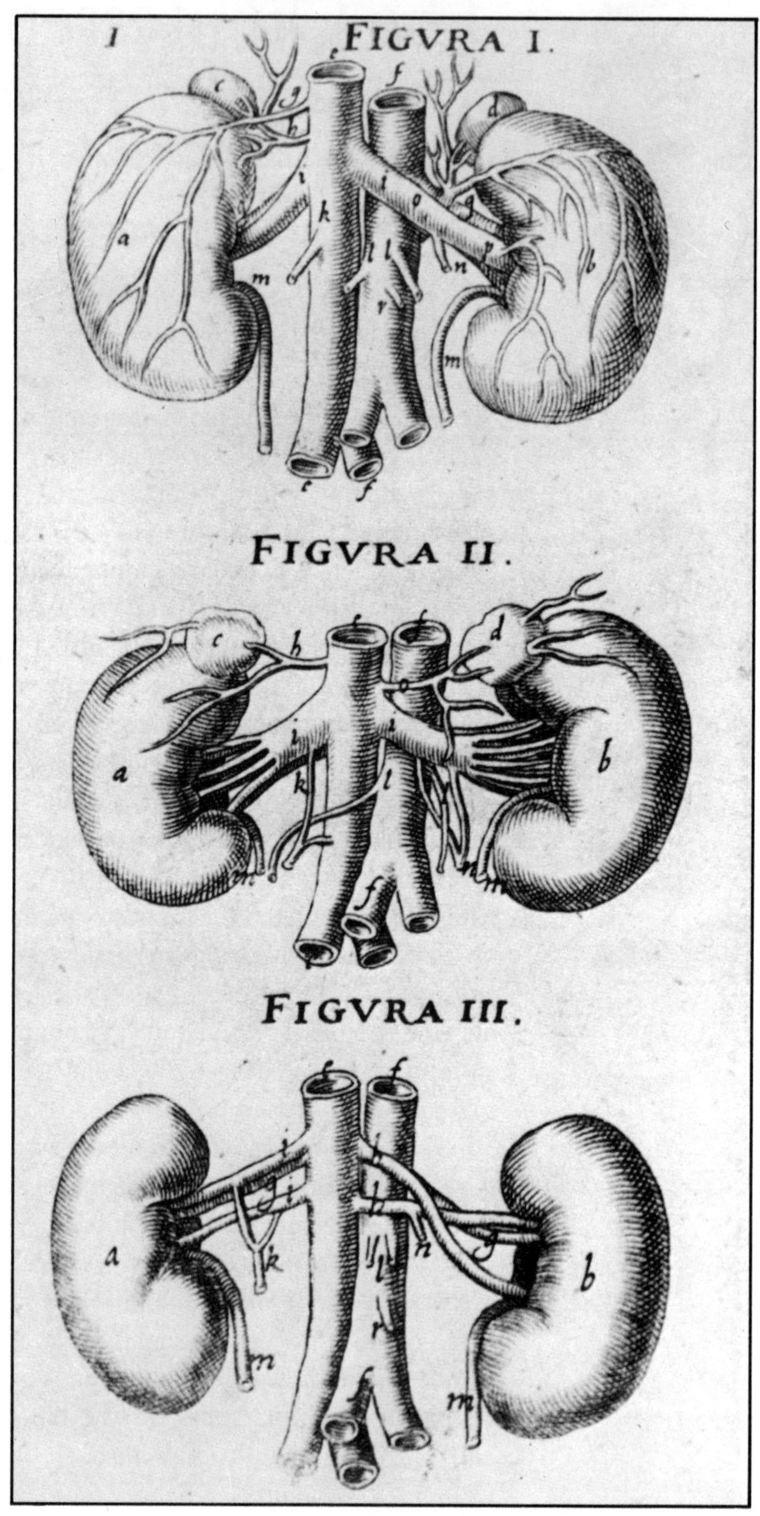

If heavy sweating during exercise has depleted salt and water from the body, then less than usual is lost into the urine. Conversely, if we drink a lot of liquid or eat highly salted foods, then that extra quantity is rapidly excreted. The net result of these compensatory responses is to maintain a constant amount of salt and water within the body fluids that bath the cells.

The regulation of salt and water losses into the urine is under the control of two separate hormones. Whenever the blood level of sodium falls, the adrenal gland liberates a substance called aldosterone. Aldosterone activates specialist pumps in the walls of the kidney tubules, which pump salt back into the blood.

When the amount of water in the body falls, another substance, antidiuretic hormone, is released from the pituitary gland at the base of the brain. This hormone opens up holes in the cells lining the tubules, so water can be reabsorbed more easily.

Some people who have head injuries suffer damage to their pituitary glands. They cannot release any antidiuretic hormone, so urine production rises from the normal one or two litres per day to more than twenty litres. These people must drink a similar volume to replace the water lost. Imagine drinking a litre of liquid every hour, day and night.

In other cases, tumours of the adrenal gland can cause excessive quantities of aldosterone to be released. The result of this deficiency, traditionally called Conn's disease, after the physician who first described it, is an accumulation of excess salt and water in the body, with a rise in blood pressure.

When salt and water are freely available, the body can survive without either aldosterone or antidiuretic hormone. On the other hand, when salt or drinking water are scarce, then these hormones are absolutely vital for survival.

Unfortunately for people who live in arid regions, however, even the release of massive amounts of antidiuretic hormone cannot totally prevent loss of body water in the urine. Metabolic wastes must be continually removed from the body so they do not poison the cells. These wastes must be dissolved in order to be excreted, and half a litre of water is the minimum volume that will dissolve all the wastes produced over a day. So at least this much urine will be produced, even if no water has been drunk at all.

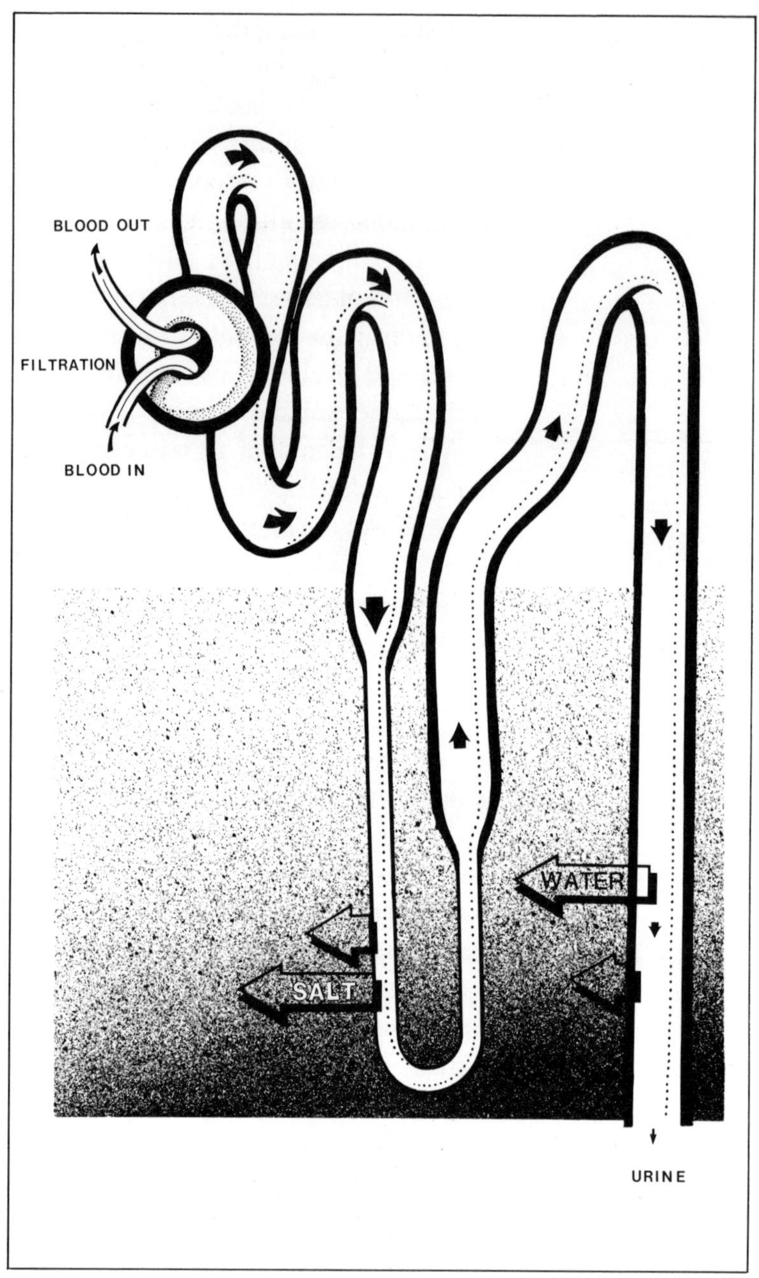

Each kidney contains millions of individual nephrons, which serve to filter the blood and to recycle essential components like salt and water. This stylised picture of one nephron shows the processes involved. After salt-containing fluid is filtered out of the bloodstream in the glomerulus, almost all the salt is selectively reabsorbed from the nephron loop, with a consequent rise in osmotic pressure in the surrounding tissue spaces, here shown as stippling. The osmotic pressure attracts water molecules out of the final portion of the nephron tubule, thus concentrating the urine.

Normally, between one and two litres of urine is formed each day, and as mentioned above, daily urine production in the absence of antidiuretic hormone may be twenty litres. But the amount that is filtered from the bloodstream into the kidney tubules over the same period is more than 200 litres. It is clear, therefore, that even without help from hormones, the kidney has an extraordinary ability to concentrate urine.

This ability is due to two things: the fact that salt particles attract water, and the fact that different parts of the tubules have very different permeabilities to salt and to water.

Each kidney tubule contains a hairpin shaped loop that dips down towards the pale centre of the kidney. Here, the tubule walls contain holes through which salt is pumped out of the tubular fluid into the surrounding tissue spaces. Because these holes are too small for water molecules to follow the salt, the system acts like a sieve, and the concentration of salt around the loop becomes far higher than it is inside the tubule.

The finale segments of the tubules, which drain urine into the base of the kidney, run close alongside the hairpin loops, so they are also surrounded by a high salt concentration. But now the tubule wall contains larger holes, so water can easily pass across it. As fluid moves through this final part of the tubule, almost all the water is sucked out by the high salt concentration outside, and reabsorbed into the bloodstream. All that is left behind is a small volume of very concentrated urine.

To keep body composition constant, we need to be able to detect when we need to drink water, as well as to stop it being lost. The most important trigger for thirst is a rise in the concentration of dissolved substances in the blood. The injection of a concentrated salt solution into the bloodstream acts on the brain to produce a sensation of thirst, even when the amount of water in the body is normal.

But there seem to be additional ways in which body water content can be monitored. A thirsty person will drink a certain amount and then stop, even though the water has not had time to be absorbed into the blood. Physiologists think that there may be sensing devices in the stomach wall, which measure the volume of water swallowed.

Usually, the amount of salt lost from the body is easily replaced in food. A salt appetite is therefore much less important than a thirst for water. But there is no doubt that salt appetite does exist. Often, the amounts of salt eaten are many times greater than that which is needed. In Australia, the average daily

Filtration of the blood takes place in the outer layer of the kidney. Here two of the glomeruli where this process occurs are marked with arrows. Each is filled with a network of capillaries, from which fluid leaks into the surrounding space that comprises the head of the nephron tubule. A stylised view of this structure is seen on the left hand side of the previous illustration. Around the glomeruli are cross-sections of the nephron tubules in which the urine is formed and concentrated.

intake is about twenty times more than that required to replace losses in sweat and urine.

We know that some varieties of laboratory rat develop high blood pressure, or hypertension, when they are fed salt. As well, many people who are unable to lose excess salt in their urine go on to develop hypertension. So, at least for some people, a high salt intake may lead to one of the cardiovascular problems associated with hypertension – strokes and heart attacks.

This is a good argument for not eating too much salt. But it is more complicated than just reducing the amount of salt we add to food. Many commercial foods and drinks contain sodium as a preservative as well as a flavouring. Quite large amounts of sodium are even added to bottled soda water.

As well, recent research suggests that salt appetite is determined in early childhood. Accepting a moderate salt intake may, for adults, therefore depend on learning to enjoy less highly salted dishes when we are young.

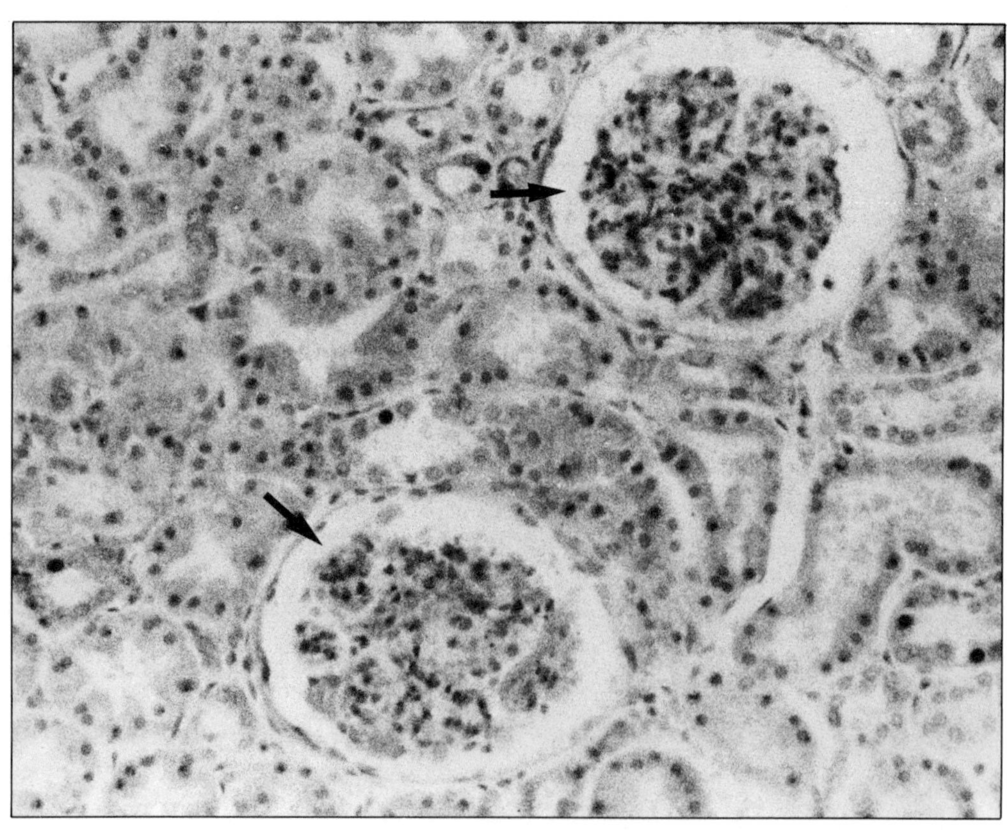

Just as salt diffuses from the bloodstream into the nephrons because its concentration is higher in the blood, other small molecules dissolved in the blood can also diffuse across the glomerulus of the kidney and be lost into the urine. Thus to keep the composition of the blood constant, it is important to control the urinary losses of these substances as well as of salt and water.

Calcium is one substance whose blood levels need to be kept within very narrow limits. Even tiny changes in the concentration of circulating calcium cause a serious malfunction of the heart and of the nervous system.

Like sodium, almost all the calcium filtered out of the bloodstream by the kidney is normally recycled by pumps in the walls of the kidney tubules. And, just as sodium reabsorption is increased by aldosterone, calcium reabsorption is also stimulated by a hormone. This one is produced from the parathyroid glands, which lie below the Adam's apple.

The parathyroid hormone also helps to maintain blood levels of calcium in two other ways. One of these is by regulating absorption of calcium from our food. The absorption process requires the presence of vitamin D. Precursors of this vitamin exist in certain foods, especially oily varieties of fish like tuna. They are also formed by the action of sunlight on the skin. But the vitamin is only active after it has been chemically transformed by parathyroid hormone. This transformation takes place in the kidney tubules, and the active vitamin D is then pumped back into the bloodstream.

Once calcium has been absorbed into the body, ninety-nine per cent of it is stored in the bones, as a lattice-work of calcium phosphate. We think of bone as a solid, permanent structure, but in fact it is continually being dissolved and remade. So calcium is continually being exchanged between blood and bone. The third way in which parathyroid hormone regulates blood calcium concentration is by speeding up the process by which bone is dissolved.

If too much of the calcium stored in bone has to be used to maintain the correct blood calcium level, then the lattice-work is weakened and the bones will fracture more easily. This sort of bone fragility, osteoporosis, is often seen in elderly people. It makes them more vulnerable to bone fractures. As well, the vertebrae of the backbone may gradually collapse, producing the bent stance which has been called 'dowager's hump'.

In children, where growth is rapid, loss of bone calcium is more serious still, causing the disease known as rickets. Here, the weight of the body causes the long bones of the legs to sag and bow outwards. The unsteady walk and fragile bones of these unfortunate children resulted in the use of the word 'ricketty' to describe unstable structures.

Calcium is more soluble in acid than in alkali. So variation in the acidity, or pH, of the blood will also affect the amount of calcium in the bloodstream. The acidity of a fluid depends on how many positively charged hydrogen ions it contains. Most hydrogen ions in the blood are 'buffered', or neutralised, by negatively charged ions such as bicarbonate. In this state, they cannot contribute to blood acidity.

But the body continually produces new hydrogen ions. They come from carbon dioxide produced in the cells, and by digestion of the proteins in food. So it is essential to have a mechanism for removing these ions from the body altogether.

Once again, the kidney plays a central role. While sodium and calcium ions are filtered from the bloodstream at the kidney glomeruli, hydrogen ions are pumped out of the bloodstream directly into the kidney tubules. Here they are buffered by phosphate and ammonia, and passed in the urine. It is these substances that help to give urine its value as a garden fertiliser.

The buffering and excretion of acid usually maintain the pH of the body within a very narrow range, just on the alkaline side of neutral. But under some circumstances, this regulation breaks down. This leads to serious changes in cell chemistry, especially in the nervous system. For instance, prolonged crying will blow most of a baby's stores of carbon dioxide out through its lungs, making the blood more alkaline. This lowers the amount of dissolved calcium, and sensitises the nerves and muscles. So the baby may twitch, and even go into convulsions. As soon as crying stops, however, normal acidity is quickly re-established by the normal cellular production of carbon dioxide.

HIDDEN SODIUM IN OUR FOOD

We usually think of sodium as being added to food to provide a salty taste. This is the way in which we eat it most, but sodium is also added to many foodstuffs and beverages for other reasons. For instance, sodium bicarbonate makes up half the weight of baking powder, monosodium glutamate (MSG) is widely used to enhance flavours, and a variety of sodium-containing substances are common preservatives.

Sometimes the actual amount of sodium added for these reasons is very small, but it is a good idea to at least be aware that it is there. Many labels on packaged food now use additive code numbers instead of specifying the additives by name. Here are common additives that contain sodium:*

201 sodium sorbate
221–223 sodium sulphites
250 sodium nitrite
251 sodium nitrate
262 sodium acetate
281 sodium propionate
301 sodium ascorbate
325 sodium lactate
331 sodium citrate
335 sodium tartrate
339 sodium phosphates
350 sodium malates
401 sodium alginate
466 sodium carboxymethylcellulose
481 sodium stearoyl lactylate
500 sodium carbonates
541 sodium aluminium phosphate
554 sodium aluminium silicate
621 monosodium glutamate
627 sodium guanylate
631 sodium inosinate

People who wish to avoid excessive sodium intake should be cautious about excessive intake of many prepared products. Here are some examples of common products that contain a lot of sodium. An ideal moderate-sodium diet should not contain more than about six grams per day.

The equivalent of one gram of common salt is consumed in:

100 gm of	*salami* *OR ham* *OR smoked or pickled fish* *OR salted butter or margarine* *OR self-raising flour*
100–200 gm of	*cheese*
200 gm of	*canned fish* *OR normal bread*

**(A complete list of code numbers for approved food additives, compiled by the National Health and Medical Research Council, is available from pharmacists, hospital dieticians and Community Health Services.)*

Chapter Eight

Keeping a Cool Head

If a cup of coffee is left sitting around, it cools down rapidly. This is because heat diffuses from the hot drink into the cooler surrounding air. Put the cup in a hot oven, and it gains heat from its surrounding environment. Human beings, like the cup of coffee, will lose or gain heat depending on the temperature of their surroundings. But, if one measures the temperature deep inside the human body, it is seen to remain almost constant, regardless of very large changes in the temperature outside. This capacity for maintenance of a constant body temperature, or 'homeothermy', is essential to the survival of man and many other animals.

Normal human body temperature is usually said to be 37°C, or 98·4°F, but this is not really accurate. Each day, our temperatures fluctuate by up to one and a half degrees Celsius because of changes in body heat production. Body temperature is lowest early in the morning and highest in the evening, and one reason for jet lag is because this temperature fluctuation becomes out of step with the new time zone.

Over the two weeks that follow ovulation, increased hormone production stimulates body heat production, and raises body temperature in women by about a further half a degree. The temperature rise is used to identify the day on which ovulation occurs, for calculation of the 'safe period' in the rhythm method of birth control.

In spite of these slow variations, however, the temperature inside any normal person varies from moment to moment by much less than one degree. Why is it important that body temperature is kept relatively high and very constant? The first reason is that all the functions of the body are driven by chemical processes, and that the rate of any chemical reaction depends on

Our body temperatures vary depending on the time of day by up to 1·5° Celsius.

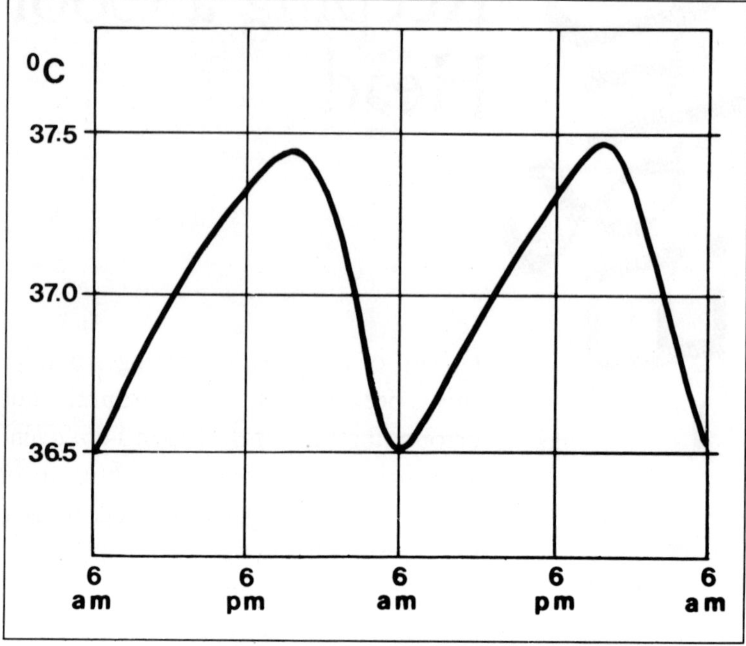

temperature. Within limits, therefore, the higher the body temperature the higher the efficiency of body chemistry. The second reason is that brain cells are extremely sensitive to changes in temperature, and, therefore, an animal that lives on its wits needs to keep its brain temperature very constant.

The physiological mechanisms that allow such a fine degree of temperature regulation are very similar to the mechanisms in an air-conditioning system. With these systems, there is a thermometer inside the room, a thermostat that can be set to a particular value and a device which heats or cools the air flowing into the room. When air temperature varies from the value set on the thermostat, this device is activated in order to heat or cool the air, and restore the set temperature.

In the case of the body, the thermostat is represented by a group of nerve cells that lie in the centre of the brain. As the primary consideration is to maintain brain temperature at a constant value, it is not surprising that the body's main thermometer is also in the brain, where a group of specialised heat-sensitive nerve cells constantly monitor blood temperature. When these cells inform the thermostat of a change in blood temperature, compensatory mechanisms change the amount of

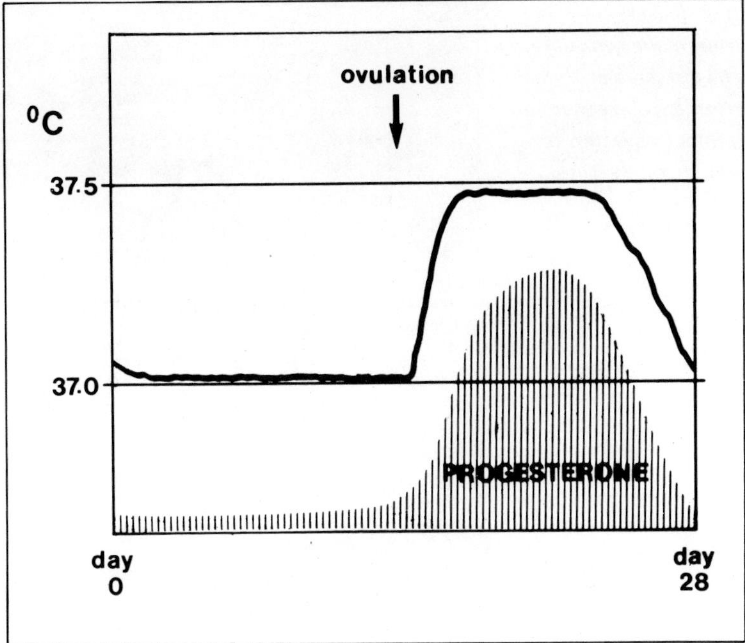

The hormone progesterone resets the body's thermostat upwards. This knowledge can be used by women to determine the day of the menstrual cycle on which ovulation has occurred.

heat produced by the body, and the rate at which it is lost into the surroundings.

Heat is produced by the normal chemical processes that make up our metabolism, so changes in metabolic rate will alter body heat production. The most easily seen example of this is the increased metabolic activity that occurs in muscles when you are cold: the process we know as shivering. Heat loss can be regulated in two ways. Altering the amount of blood that runs through the skin will alter the rate at which heat is moved from the core of the body to its edges. So, when you are cold there is little skin blood flow and the skin appears pale, and when you are hot the skin is flushed by the large amount of blood flowing through it. Sweating is the second way of changing heat loss. When you are overheated, as much as one litre of water and five grams of salt is lost from the body each hour, so it is not surprising that people in hot places need a large intake of these substances.

Think about a person sitting in a room which is maintained at a comfortable temperature – say 22°C. We know that the temperature deep inside the person will be about 37°C and that the temperature just outside the person's skin must be 22°C. As

Human body temperature normally remains constant, regardless of the environmental temperature to which we are exposed.

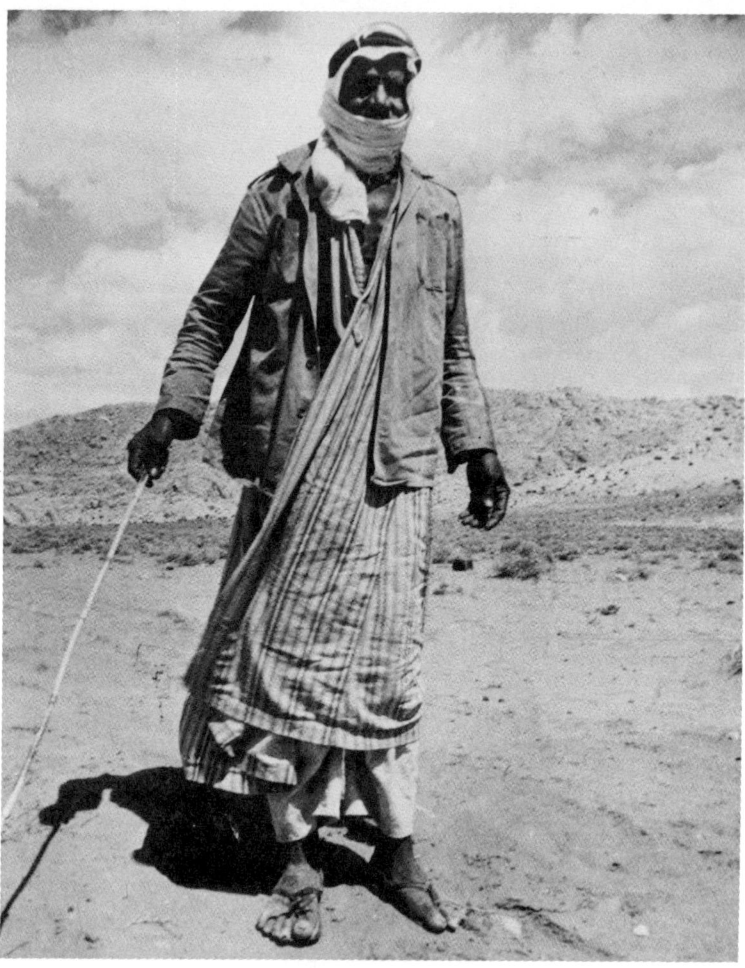

the surrounding air is colder than the person, there must be continual diffusion of heat from the body to the air, and the parts of the body that are thinnest and furthest away from the body core, such as the fingers and toes, might cool down considerably before there is any change in brain temperature. In these circumstances there would therefore be a large amount of body heat lost before the brain thermometer detected it, and a correspondingly large amount of extra energy needed to restore normal temperature.

In real life, this problem is partly solved by the existence of a second set of thermometer nerve cells, which monitor skin temperature. The rate at which the body cools down depends on the temperature of the surrounding environment, and environmental temperature will affect skin temperature. Information on skin temperature therefore allows the brain to anticipate whether heat loss is occurring fast enough to decrease temperature deep in the body, and to trigger appropriate compensatory processes before this has happened. So skin cooling or skin warming, as well as changes in blood temperature, can result in alterations of body heat production or exchange with the environment.

Paradoxically, it is the information received by the brain from these skin temperature receptors, rather than the temperature deep within the body, that determines whether we feel warm or cold. In fact, provided that the skin is kept warm, dangerous falls in body temperature can occur without any warning signals. For instance, consumption of alcohol increases skin temperature by relaxing the skin blood vessels, thus allowing more skin blood flow. This produces a sensation of warmth, even when the body as a whole is becoming cold.

In a cold environment, alcohol consumption has another effect as well. As discussed earlier in this chapter, the rate at which heat leaves the body is altered by the amount of skin blood flow. So, if the blood flow is increased by alcohol, this increases the rate of body cooling as well as maintaining a misleading feeling of warmth. This is why alcohol consumption is not advisable for people such as mountain walkers.

Heat exchange between the body and the outside world is regulated by complex behavioural responses as well as by the more basic physiological mechanisms that we have been dealing with up until now. The postural attitudes adopted by people when they are cold or hot are so well known that their practical importance is often ignored. Think about your unconscious reactions to standing in a cold wind: you may hunch your shoulders and hug yourself, you may clap your hands or stamp your feet. All these actions are valuable in body heat conservation – the posture adopted minimises the exposed surface area of the body, thus reducing heat loss, while the extra muscular activity generates metabolic heat. Compare your reactions to cold with those you have to a roasting summer day. You are likely to move more slowly (so reducing heat production), and you certainly will not adopt a huddled posture. Rather, you are likely to maximise the exposed skin area by keeping your arms away from your body and holding your fingers loose (so increasing heat loss).

You can see that the regulation of body temperature involves a number of interlinking mechanisms. There are, however, some even more sophisticated ways in which the body can cope with climatic extremes. These extra mechanisms serve to reduce the metabolic demands imposed by high or low environmental temperatures, and expand enormously the range of environments in which humans can live.

Maintaining a constant body temperature is an expensive process; the mechanisms for both heat loss and heat gain require a lot of metabolic energy. Climates that are very hot or very cold therefore impose severe demands on our energy stores. But we have evolved some rather clever design features by which this expense can be minimised.

One of these is based on a principle termed counter-current exchange. Engineers have known for many years that, if two streams of fluid at different temperatures flow past each other in opposite directions, heat is transferred from the hotter fluid to the cooler. The blood supplying our hands and feet travels in arteries that lie in the centre of the limbs, but it can return to the body in either of two sets of veins. One lies close to the arteries, the other close to the skin surface. The proportion of blood flowing in each is regulated by nerves that shut off one or other set of veins.

When the brain detects a fall in body temperature, blood returning from the hands and feet is directed into the central veins, and there is countercurrent movement of heat from venous to arterial blood, cooling the blood reaching the hands and feet and retaining heat within the body core. It is easy to see, therefore, why when we are in a cool environment our fingers and toes feel so cold. By contrast, when a rise in body temperature occurs, blood returning from the extremities is diverted totally to the surface veins, where it is able to lose heat into the air and so help to cool the body core.

An expedition to Central Australia led by Sir Stanton Hicks in 1934 found an entirely different sort of trick was used by the nomadic Aboriginals in order to reduce the amount of energy needed for temperature control. A group of Aboriginals and a group of white scientists slept under similar conditions on a winter's night in the desert, where the air temperature was close to zero. The scientists felt very cold, but managed to maintain their body temperatures by violent shivering. The Aboriginals, by contrast, did not feel cold and did not shiver. During the night their body temperatures fell by several degrees. In other words, they were able to turn off their central heating systems while they were asleep, and so save energy. This seems to be a sensible economy in a population with a traditionally low nutritional intake, and the same pattern has been described in other nomadic societies. What we don't know is whether such a specialised adaptation can occur in any group of people subjected to the appropriate conditions for a long time, or whether it is genetically determined.

The phenomena that I have talked about so far can all be regarded as economic measures to cut the costs of temperature regulation, but the picture would be incomplete without mentioning one further important mechanism which, in terms of energy expenditure, is a very expensive one. We know that exposure to cold causes a reduction in skin blood flow, and pale skin. Yet when one is exposed to very low temperatures the ears, nose, fingers and toes become visibly flushed, showing that their blood flow must be high. All these areas of the body have very large surface areas compared with their internal volumes, which means that they cool down very rapidly. If the surrounding environment is cold enough, they may actually freeze. This is avoided by the presence under the skin of specialised blood vessels, which open when the temperature of the skin falls to just above freezing point. A large increase in blood flow therefore occurs, and causes the skin to rewarm.

A British expedition to the Himalayas in the winter of 1961 witnessed a dramatic example of how effective this protective device can be. At an altitude of 5000 metres, with the snow at temperatures well below freezing point, the team met at Nepalese pilgrim. This man had no gloves or footwear, and no sleeping bag. He stayed with the expedition for several days, and showed no signs whatsoever of discomfort, or of damage to his hands or feet.

Unfortunately, cold flushing is not so effective in people who are not habituated to cold conditions. Those of us who enjoy an occasional skiing trip, or spend a holiday in the northern winter, still need to help our temperature regulating systems along with caps, scarves, gloves and socks in order to protect ourselves from the damaging effects of the environment.

HYPERTHERMIA
causes, dangers and treatment

Causes – *Inadequate fluid and salt replacement during exercise.*
Insufficient heat loss in sweat because of high atmospheric humidity or too much clothing, or poor sweat production due to drugs or sickness.
Resetting of brain thermostat by infection.

Dangers – *Loss of body fluids due to heavy sweating causes drop in blood volume and blood pressure.*
High temperature causes protein coagulation in cells of brain.

Treatment – *Collapse during exercise is almost always because of fluid loss: provide up to 1 litre cool (not ice-cold) water with 1 tablespoon of table salt per litre.*
Move person into shade, and remove clothing so as to increase evaporation of sweat. Sponging with cool (not ice-cold) water will help cooling.
In the rare cases where a person is dramatically hyperthermic, they should be placed in a bath of water as cold as possible.
People with mild fevers (up to 38·5°C) will feel better when treated with aspirin, but may actually get better more slowly.
At higher temperatures, use aspirin and cooling sponges.

HYPOTHERMIA
causes, dangers and treatment

Causes – *In well-nourished adults, hypothermia occurs only when heat loss from the body is very rapid, because of immersion in cold water or because the insulating effect of clothing has been reduced by wetting it. Children are more at risk, because they can't store as much heat in their bodies. Old people are also at risk, because they lose heat more quickly.*

Dangers – *All the dangerous effects of cooling are due to the fact that electrical activity in nerves and muscles is slowed down. Body temperatures only a couple of degrees below normal produce incoordination, stumbling and fumbling. At 31°C, consciousness is lost. At 25°C, the heart stops.*

Treatment – *The crucial thing is to stop heat loss, by placing a good layer of insulation around the victim and providing a shelter from wind or rain. After this is done, a source of conducted heat (hot water bottles, a dry dog, another person) can be placed inside the insulation. If you have to carry an unconscious or injured person who is hypothermic, don't tilt them head-up, because the blood flow to the brain will fall.*

Chapter Nine

The New and the Old

Perhaps the most dramatic example of biological complexity is the normal development of an organism such as a human being from a single fertilised cell. Not only does this cell divide so that it forms many different types of tissue with highly specialised functions, but extraordinarily precise connections are laid down between the components of these tissues, finally resulting in an individual at once identical to and subtly different from its parents.

The basis for this developmental precision is probably the single most important question being asked in biology today, as it involves understanding the very basis for our existence as a species. For those of us who work at the interface between pure and applied biology, finding an answer has another implication. Knowing the mechanisms that control how different cells become specialised as they mature may provide the means to treat many disorders in which the normal specialisation processes seem to have become abnormal. These include a variety of congenital defects, some cancers, and some diseases of the brain such as Alzheimer's disease and Parkinsonism.

Most of the experimental work involving nervous system development has been concerned with the interactions of muscle cells and the nerve cells that control them. As the embryo grows, cells in the developing brain and spinal cord send out sprouts towards the areas that will become the limbs and the body wall. By the time of birth, each of these nerves will have made precise contact with a particular muscle cell, so that it can perform its specific movement task. Even if a segment of spinal cord is cut out and turned around, the nerves form contacts with the correct muscles.

Such precision of growth seems to imply that each muscle

must emit a signal instructing its particular nerve to make contact, and some sort of chemical recognition is probably involved, so that the nerves can detect that they have reached an area containing potential target cells. But the large number of nerves and muscles present in the body makes it unlikely that different chemical signals exist for every single one. As well, at the time that the nerves arrive at their destinations the muscle cells have not yet appeared.

Much of the precision of contact is likely to be due to the strict sequence of development in different parts of the body, so that the interaction of each group of nerve and muscle cells occurs just at the right stage of their growth.

The survival of both nerves and muscles depends on these contacts being established. A developing limb that does not

Female Emigration
TO
AUSTRALIA.
COMMITTEE:
EDWARD FORSTER, Esq. Chairman.
SAMUEL HOARE, Esq.
JOHN TAYLOR, Esq.
THOMAS LEWIN, Esq.
S. H. STERRY, Esq.
CHARLES HOLTE BRACEBRIDGE, Esq.
JOHN S. REYNOLDS, Esq.
JOHN PIRIE, Esq.
CAPEL CURE, Esq.
WILLIAM CRAWFORD, Esq.
CHARLES LUSHINGTON, Esq.
JOHN ABEL SMITH, Esq. M.P.
GEORGE LONG, Esq.
COLONEL PHIPPS,
NADIR BAXTER, Esq.
CAPTAIN DANIEL PRING, R.N.
The Committee for promoting the Emigration
OF
Single Women
To AUSTRALIA, acting under the Sanction of His Majesty's Secretary of State for the Colonies, HEREBY GIVE NOTICE, That
THE SPLENDID TEAK-BUILT SHIP
"David Scott," of 773 Tons Register,
Carrying an experienced Surgeon, and a respectable Person and his Wife as Superintendents to secure the Comfort and Protection of the Emigrants during the Voyage, will sail from
GRAVESEND
On Thursday 10th of July next,
(Beyond which day she will on no account be detained) direct for
SYDNEY.
Single Women and Widows of good Character, from 15 to 30 Years of Age, desirous of bettering their Condition by Emigrating to that healthy and highly prosperous Colony, where the number of Females compared with the entire Population is greatly deficient, and where consequently from the great demand for Servants, and other Female Employments, the Wages are comparatively high, may obtain a Passage
On payment of FIVE POUNDS only.
Those who are unable to raise even that Sum here, may, when approved by the Committee, go without any Money Payment whatever, as their Notes of Hand will be taken, payable in the Colony within a reasonable time after their arrival, when they have acquired the means to do so: in both cases the Parties will have the advantage of the Government Grant in aid of their Passage.
The Females who proceed by this Conveyance will be taken care of on their first Landing at Sydney. They will find there a List of the various Situations to be obtained, and of the Wages offered, and will be perfectly free to make their own Election; they will not be bound to any person, or subjected to any restraint, but will be, to all intents and purposes, perfectly free to act and decide for themselves.
Females in the Country who may desire to avail themselves of the important advantages thus offered them, should apply by Letter to "The Emigration Committee, London," under Cover addressed to "The UNDER SECRETARY OF STATE, COLONIAL DEPARTMENT, LONDON." It will be necessary that the Application be accompanied by a Certificate of Character from the Resident Minister of the Parish, or from some other respectable persons to whom the Applicant may be known; but the Certificate of the Resident Minister is in all cases most desirable. Such Females as may find it expedient may, when approved by the Committee as fit persons to go by this Conveyance, be boarded temporarily in London, prior to Embarkation, on Payment of 7s. per Week.
All Applications made under cover in the foregoing manner, or personally, will receive early Answers, and all necessary Information, by applying to
JOHN MARSHALL, Agent to the Committee, 26, Birchin Lane, Cornhill, London.
EDWARD FORSTER, Chairman.
NOTE.—The Committee have the satisfaction to state that of 217 Females who went out by the "Bussorah Merchant," 180 obtained good Situations within three Days of their Landing, and the remainder were all well placed within a few Days, under the advice of a Ladies' Committee, formed in the Colony expressly to aid the Females on their arrival.
LONDON, 1st May, 1834
By Authority:

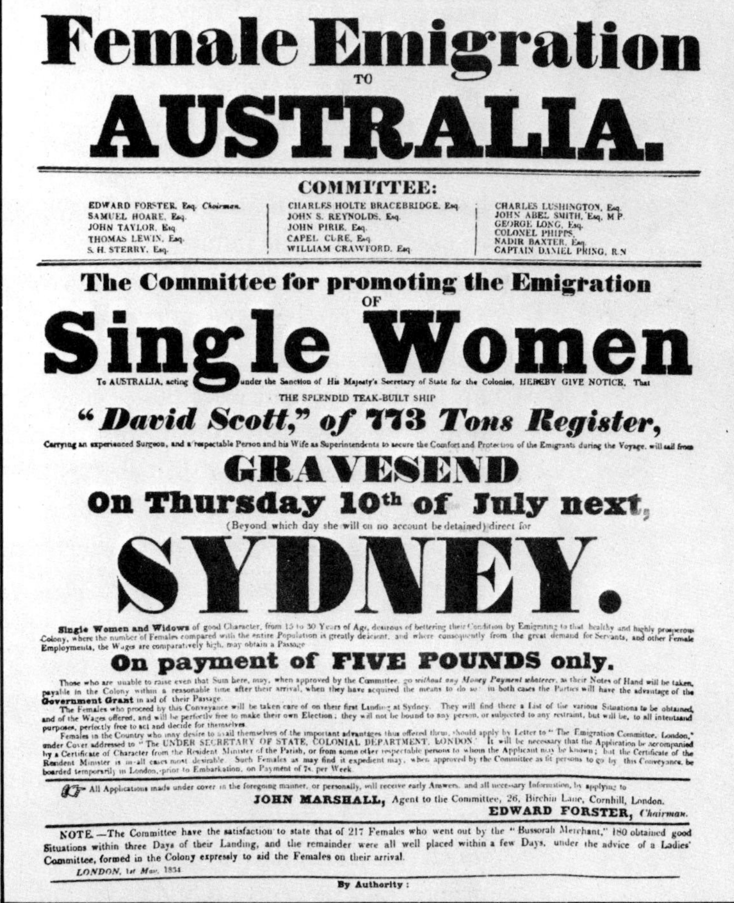

The migration of people from one part of the world to another has had important effects on the genetic composition of communities. Emigration poster c. 1834. La Trobe Library.

receive any nerves fails to mature: drugs such as thalidomide that cause limb deformities probably act by inhibiting this process. Conversely, the removal of the developing limb before the nerves arrive results in death of the nerve cells themselves.

The interaction between nerves and their target cells is rather different for the developing internal organs. Unlike the nerves supplying our various limb muscles, which all use the same chemical neurotransmitter, the nerve cells that supply various organs in the abdomen, such as the adrenal gland and the intestine, use separate neurotransmitters. During early development, these nerves can be persuaded to grow into areas that they do not normally enter, by turning around the segment of the nervous system from which they are sprouting. This results in the formation of connections with organs that they would not normally supply. Remarkably, the nerves now release the neurotransmitter substance appropriate to the new target organ, and not to the one that they would normally contact. So, for these nerves, the way in which they mature is clearly determined by a signal emitted from the target tissue.

Physiologists Stephen Kuffler, John Nicholls and Bob Martin have suggested that the task of trying to use findings like these to comprehend the human brain may be analogous to analysing how the postal system works. Sending a letter from (say) Australia to England can be broken down into many steps, each involving only a few instructions. The letter writer must know where to post the letter, but does not need to know how it gets to the post office; the central mail sorter in Sydney is not concerned with the details of the British postal service, and so on. By working through these small, apparently isolated steps, the whole process may at last be revealed.

This analogy also highlights how easy it is to ask futile questions in biology. For instance, we cannot find out anything useful about how the system works by asking whether the Sydney mail sorter knows the English postman, or by finding out the name of the aeroplane that carries the letter to London.

As well as the precise instructions that direct the development of the body before birth, other instructions determine how much we continue to grow after this time. A look at the proportions of medieval buildings, and the displays in European

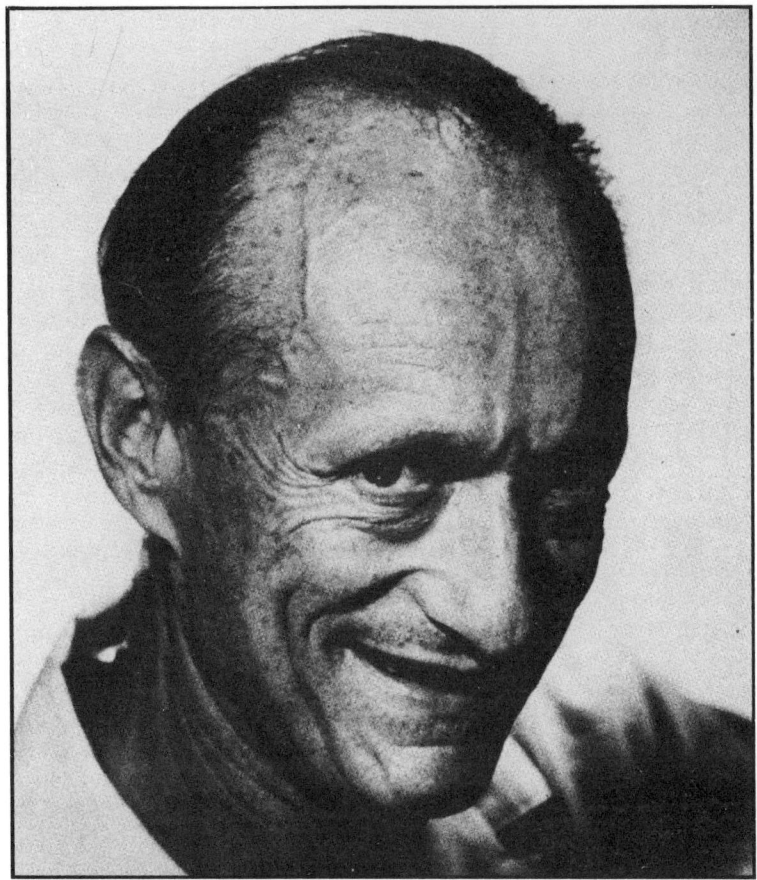

Stephen Kuffler (1913–1980) was responsible for shaping many of our ideas about the development of the nervous system.

museums, shows dramatically how much the size of the human body has changed over the last thousand years. Few modern men could fit into the suits of armour typical of the Middle Ages; not many of us can walk through the doorways of a medieval castle without stooping.

These changes in height have been quite well documented for some populations. The average English foot soldier of medieval times stood about 160 cm tall; by 1900 this had increased to 170 cm, and by 1960 by another 4 cm. Thousands of years would be required for natural selection to cause such a large change, so normal evolutionary processes cannot be implicated. How then can this continued growth be explained?

One explanation that has been frequently put forward is the effect of improved nutrition on body growth. The increased mixing of genetic material with increased travel between different

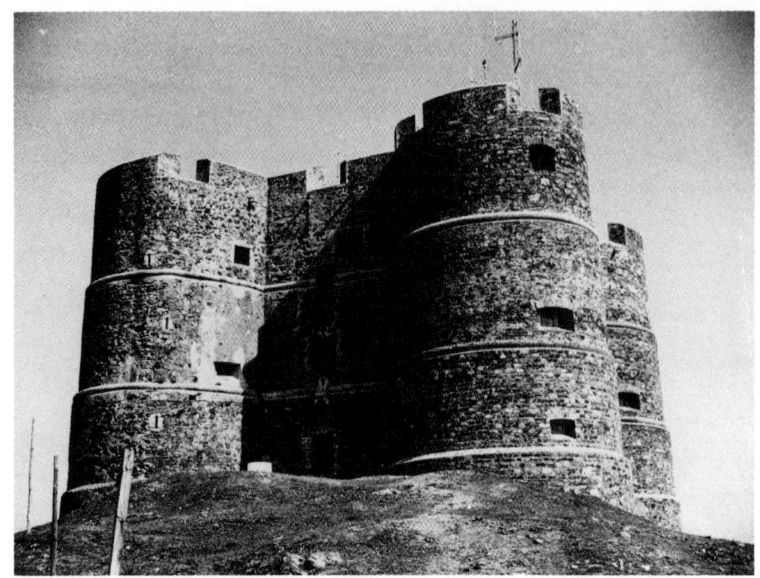

The smallness of the doorways found in European castles of the middle ages had a partly defensive basis, but it also reminds us that the people of those times were considerably smaller in stature than we are nowadays.

parts of the world is also probably involved. For instance, the inhabitants of northern Europe are, in general, taller in stature than the inhabitants of southern Europe, so intermarriage between the two populations tends to increase body height in the southern population.

Some scientists, however, believe that adaptive evolutionary forces may also be acting, despite the time scales being far too short for traditional natural selection to be effective. By this theory, habitual changes in lifestyle from generation to generation might result in modification of the genetic code and so cause the inheritance of physical changes. Such adaptations apparently can occur. For example, the changes in Western diet over the last few hundred years have already been associated with the functional loss of some of our grinding teeth – the so-called wisdom teeth.

If this evolutionary theory holds true as a general rule, then we can predict what our descendants might look like. Increased reliance on computerisation and mental, rather than physical, approaches to work will increase the size of certain parts of the brain, and the absence of tough food will decrease the size of the jaw bone. Both these factors will change the head shape, enlarging the top of the skull and shrinking the chin. At the same time, decreased emphasis on physical activity at work and in leisure pursuits will produce a dwindling of muscle and bone bulk in the limbs. The resulting tadpole-like person would be remarkably like some of the interplanetary monsters seen in science fiction comics: probably a practicable adaptation to circumstances, but somehow not a great tribute to the history of human civilisation.

In contrast to these imponderables, the factors that regulate body size within one generation are well described. Retardation of growth can occur through four different types of deficiency. There may be inadequate food intake in general, resulting in lack of all dietary constituents needed for tissue nourishment. In developing countries, an even more common problem is selective deficiency in the intake of protein, the amino acids of which are necessary for building new cells. In children, an inadequate protein diet interferes with the ability of the capillaries to retain water in the bloodstream, so it tends to leak out into the abdominal cavity, producing the characteristic pot-belly that we associate with malnutrition.

Even if food intake is sufficient, hormonal influences are also needed to ensure that growth occurs. A thyroid-stimulating hormone acts on the thyroid gland to stimulate protein synthesis, while a growth hormone stimulates the growth of cartilage and bone. Both of these hormones are released from the pituitary gland, situated at the base of the brain just above the roof of the mouth. Tumours of the pituitary gland in childhood, resulting in abnormal amounts of hormone release, will also result in abnormal growth patterns. Nevertheless, there is a very wide normal range of growth rates, as well as a wide range of normal heights at adulthood. So most children who seem at one age to be very short or very tall, relative to their peers, will catch up or be caught up with, over the next few years.

As well as the continuing increase in stature, another striking characteristic of modern Western society is a gradual but progressive increase in the average age of the population. Over the next twenty years, the number of people over sixty will double. The elderly section of the community therefore represents an increasingly important focus of health care, and understanding the mechanisms that make up the ageing process is becoming more and more essential.

Some of the cells in our bodies, like nerve and muscle cells,

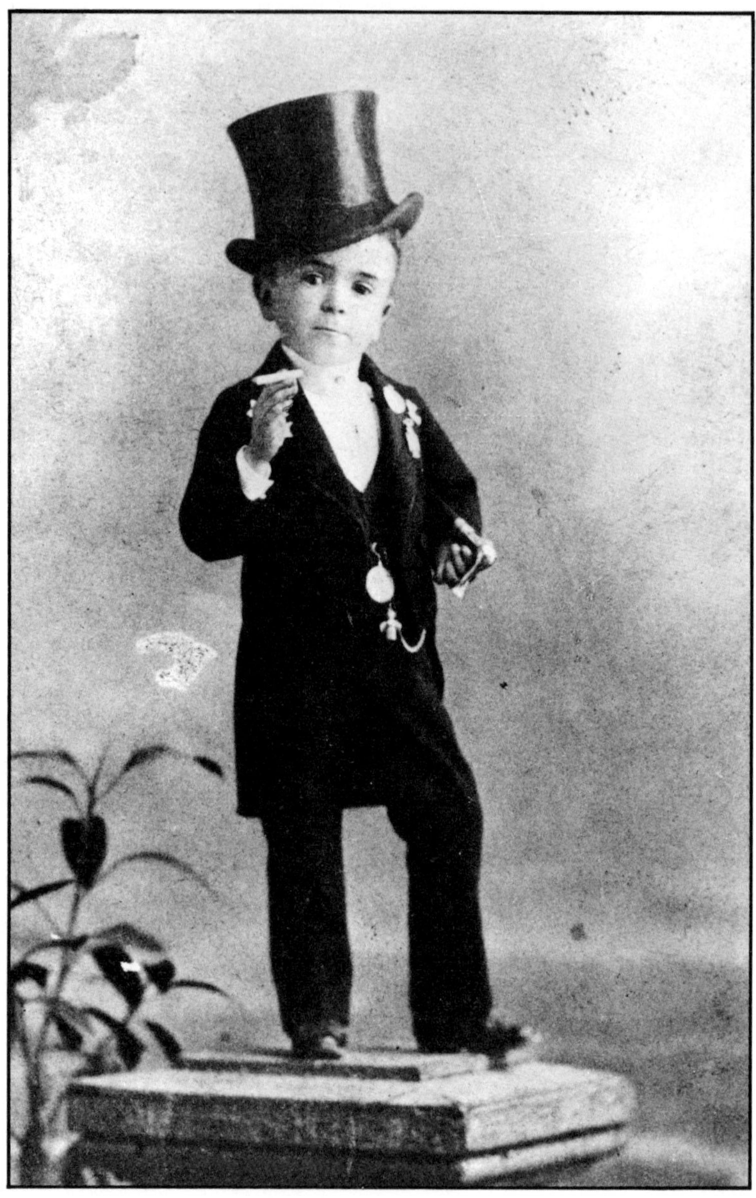

Childhood deficiency of certain hormones can result in a dramatic reduction in the amount of growth that occurs. General Tom Thumb in Western Australia, *1882. La Trobe Library.*

which do highly specialised jobs, are hardly manufactured at all after birth. Other, less specialised, cells, which carry out the routine tasks of holding the body together, fighting infections and transporting foodstuffs and waste products, continue to multiply all our lives. What we recognise as ageing is probably the gradual loss of this ability to form new cells. One experimental finding that supports this view is the fact that, in a tissue culture, cells will divide only a certain number of times before they stop, and the number of divisions is proportional to the normal lifespan of the species from which the cells were taken.

Biologists working on ageing (gerontologists) have explained this manufacturing shutdown by a number of alternative theories. The first of these is that faults develop in the DNA strands carrying genetic information from one cell generation to the next. The second is that the body's immune system develops faults, and begins to mistake body cells for foreign invaders. A third possibility would be the exhaustion of stores of some vital nutrient. Finally, changes in the processes of cell chemistry might produce poisonous waste products and cell death.

Finding the answer to the ageing question presents two great difficulties. Even if one of the processes suggested above can be identified as occurring (and probably more than one is involved), this still may not tell us *why* it occurs. The second difficulty is a practical one: if the process being investigated takes up to fifty years to occur, then how can one study its details? Many crucial observations can be made only in a species that has a normal lifespan short enough for many generations to be studied in the investigator's own lifetime. In gerontology then, as in many other areas of biomedical research, laboratory animals play an important role in the acquisition of knowledge to help the human population.

A further complication is the variability that one sees in the ageing process between different societies. Although we still talk about 'three score years and ten' as a typical lifespan, in some rural communities like those of the Hunzas of central Asia and the Amerindians of the Andes quite a high proportion of individuals live well over 100 years.

Superficially, it seems as if this can be explained by their lifestyle: they are physically active manual labourers, they have diets that are low in animal protein and they live in low-density housing in a pollution-free and stress-free environment. Most doctors in our society would regard all those factors as predisposing to a long and healthy life. On the other hand, the Amerindians also consume, on average, three cups of rum and fifty cigarettes every day. An Australian GP is unlikely to be convinced that these habits would increase longevity!

TYPICAL NORMAL GROWTH RATES

Typical normal growth rates for girls and boys. Before birth, there is no difference between the rate of growth of the two sexes. Note the rapid growth spurt seen in boys at puberty (14–15 years), and the more gradual growth in girls, but also remember that growth in particular children may occur at quite different rates than these typical values.

	Girls		Boys	
Age	*Weight (kg)*	*Height (cm)*	*Weight (kg)*	*Height (cm)*
Birth	3.2	50	3.4	51
1 month	3.9	53	4	55
3 months	5.5	60	6	61
6 months	7.5	67	8.1	69
9 months	8.6	71	9.4	73
1 year	9.5	75	10.1	77
1.5 years	11	82	11.3	83
2 years	12.1	88	12.5	88
3 years	14.3	95	14.6	96
4 years	16.3	102	16.7	104
5 years	18.3	109	18.9	110
6 years	21	116	21	117
7 years	24	122	23	122
8 years	27	128	25	128
9 years	29	133	28	133
10 years	32	138	31	138
11 years	35	142	35	143
12 years	39	149	40	147
13 years	44	154	44	153
14 years	50	158	49	160
15 years	53	161	53	167
16 years	55	163	58	172
17 years	57	164	61	174

(Data adapted from Scientific Tables, 7th edition, Ciba-Geigy, 1970.)

Chapter Ten

Looking Outwards . . .

The eye is the most sophisticated of all the systems we have for detecting what is happening in the world around our bodies. It is extraordinarily sensitive: the light of one candle can be seen twenty-five kilometres away. It can detect very small differences in light wavelength, giving us the benefit of colour vision. It discriminates fine detail, allowing us to read small print and to focus on objects that are close or far away. And, by showing us our surroundings, it plays an important part in the control of balance.

The basic principles by which the eye works are similar to those of a camera. At the front of the eye, a convex lens focusses light rays onto the retina, and a ring of muscle fibres acts as a diaphragm to alter the amount of light that enters. This diaphragm forms the iris, and the hole through which light passes is the pupil. At the back of the eye, the light falls on sensitive nerve cells in the retina, corresponding to the photographic film of the camera.

Removed from the eye, the lens is almost spherical. But normally, it is pulled out almost flat by muscle fibres that fix it to the rim of the eyeball. When we look at an object that is close to us, these muscles relax and allow the lens to swell. This increases its power, so that light beams which originate closer to the eye can be focussed onto the retina.

There are no blood vessels inside the lens, because this would interfere with vision. So the cells in the lens centre are always slightly oxygen deficient, and die earlier than those in the outer part. The consequence is that, as we age, the lens becomes stiff and cannot swell as much when the muscles around its edge relax. This is the reason why older people find it harder to focus on close objects.

Like a camera, accurate focussing by the lens depends on a constant distance between lens and retina. To achieve this, the eyeball is filled with fluid under pressure. The fluid is filtered from the blood into the eye chamber, and then slowly drains out through spaces around the lens, into the space behind the outer covering of the eye, or cornea. In the disease called glaucoma, this drainage system becomes blocked, and pressure builds up in the eyeball. The pressure squashes blood vessels supplying the light-sensing retina, which is deprived of oxygen. So untreated glaucoma can easily lead to blindness.

The retina contains two sorts of light-sensitive cells. The 'cones', which are concentrated in the central area, can detect only bright light. The 'rods', which predominate around the margins of the retina, can detect even very dim light. In bright surroundings, the pupil is constricted, so light rays mainly hit the centre of the retina and activate the cones. But when the amount of light is too low to be detected here, the pupil opens and light reaches the more sensitive rods.

Although they are better at detecting light, the rods produce a less precise image than the cones do. The different amount of detail seen is similar to comparing a high quality photograph, where the grain size is very small, with a newspaper reproduction, which is made up of quite coarse dots of ink. So in the dark, when our vision is operating entirely through the rod system, outlines and details of objects appear blurred.

Both rod and cone cells contain light-sensitive 'photopigments', consisting of a protein molecule that is bound to a pigmented derivative of vitamin A. When these photopigments are hit by light rays, they change their shape, and this in turn causes a change in the leakiness of the cell to sodium ions. The resulting electrical message is then passed through a chain of nerve cells to the part of the brain responsible for interpreting visual messages.

The effect of light on the photopigments involves only movements of the electrical bonds that hold them together. It is therefore extremely fast, occurring in about one-million-millionth of a second. But reversal of the process relies on the chemical action of enzymes to remodel the photopigment molecule, and is very much slower. Consequently, after they respond

The explorers Burke and Wills, like many others who have tried to cross deserts, died because they could not find the regular supply of water that is essential for human survival. Natives Discovering the Body of William John Wills, the Explorer, at Cooper's Creek, June 1861, *E. M. Scott. La Trobe Library.*

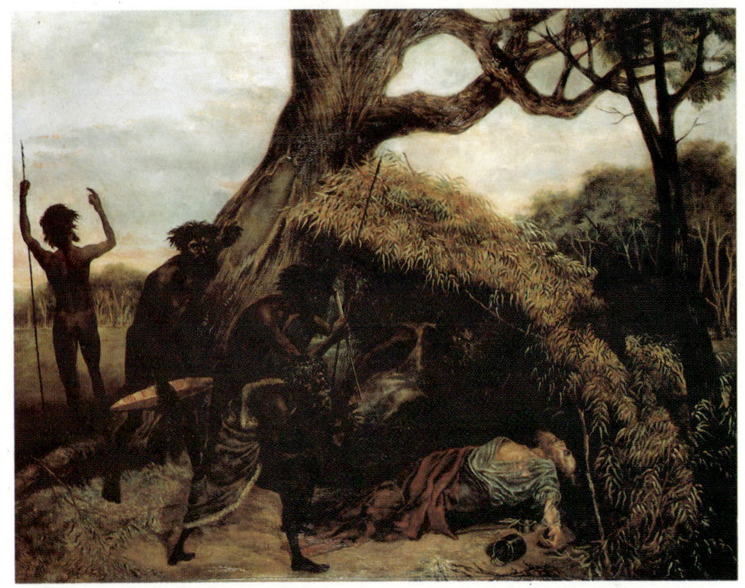

Nomadic societies which are exposed to large daily fluctuations in environmental temperature have become highly resistant to cold, allowing them to exist comfortably without protective clothing. Constitution Hill at Sunset, From Near Mrs Ranson's Public House, *J. Glover. La Trobe Library.*

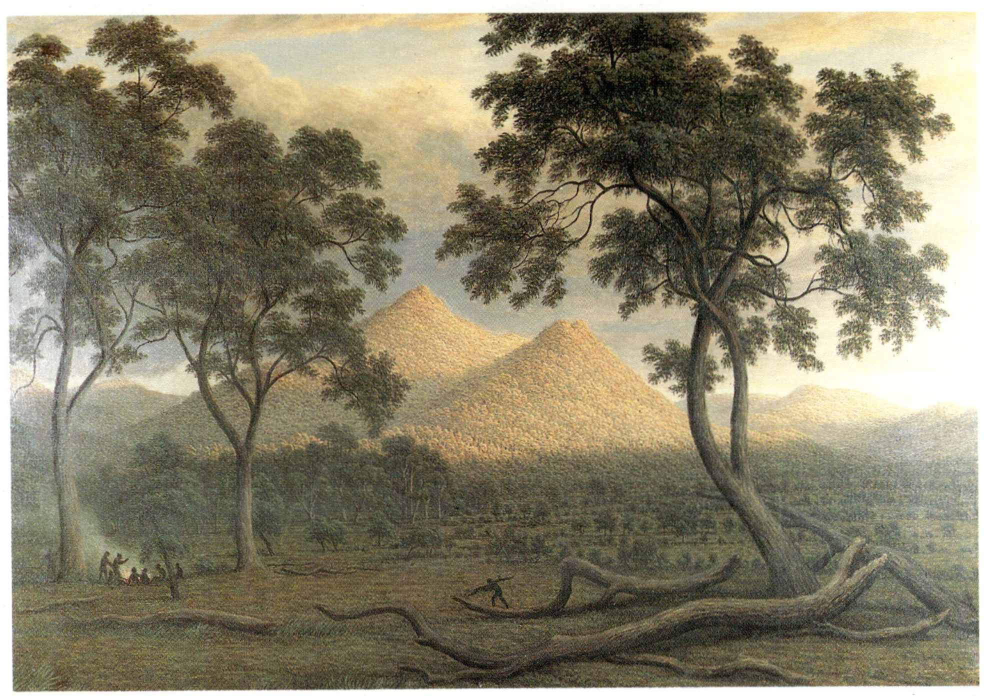

Our eyes can be deceived by some patterns. Because of the arrangement of light and dark areas, this picture looks as if there is a dark stripe down its centre.

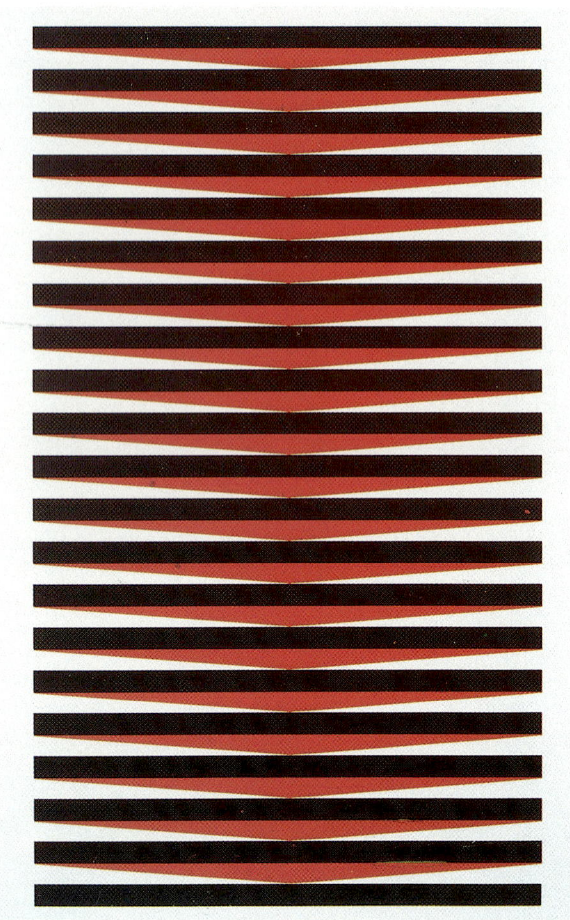

Angular motion can disturb the normal mechanisms in the ear that maintain our sense of balance, and may lead to nausea. S.S. Toroa, *A. V. Gregory. La Trobe Library.*

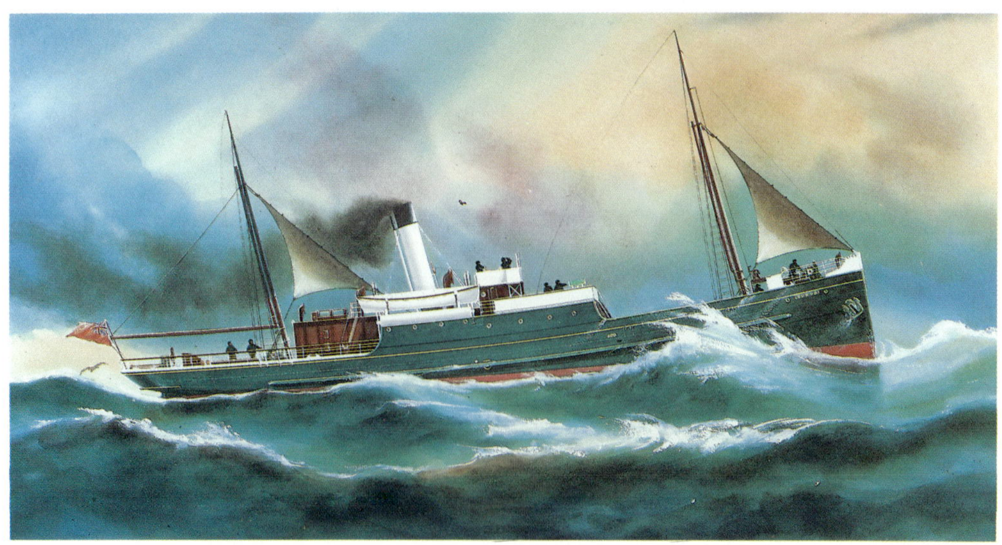

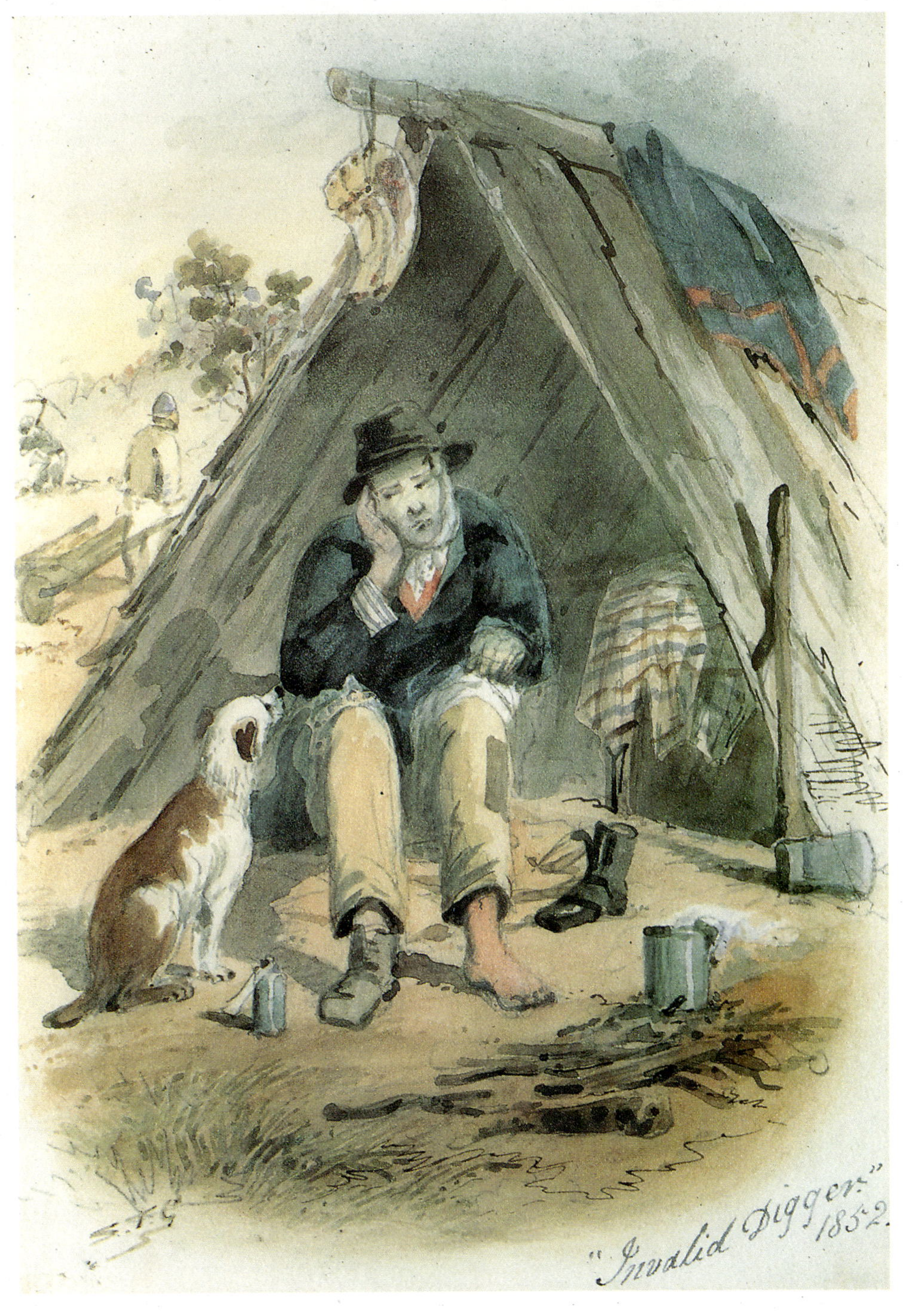

Pain is an important warning system for protection of the body. Invalid Digger, *S. T. Gill. La Trobe Library.*

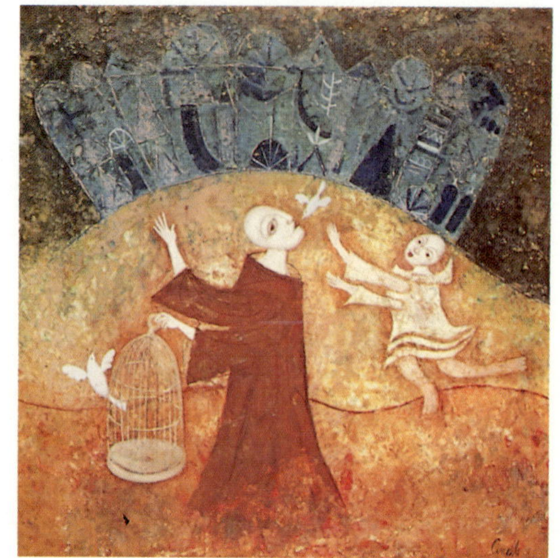

Although it is possible to identify areas of the brain responsible for many patterns of behaviour, we still know nothing about the biological processes associated with human attributes like religious faith, artistic ability and aesthetic appreciation.

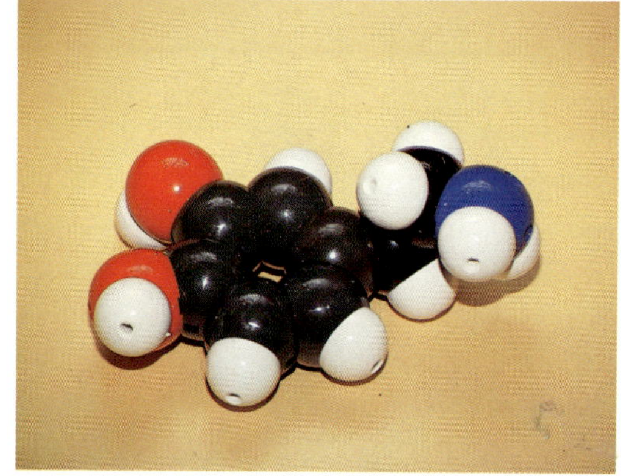

Dopamine is a molecule that has important roles as a neurotransmitter in several parts of the nervous system. Here, molecular modelling shows the composition of this substance. The white balls represent hydrogen atoms, the black carbon atoms, the red oxygen, and the blue nitrogen. The central grey structure is a benzene ring.

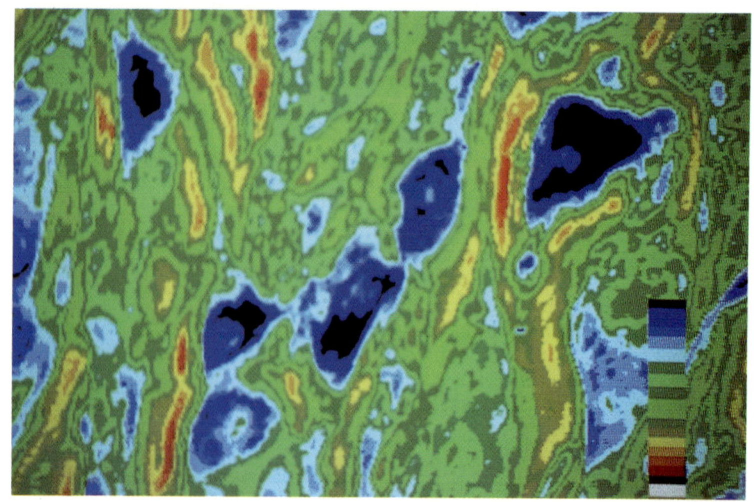

The use of computerised technologies are helping to unravel some of the mysteries of the nervous system. Here, a computer has been used to demonstrate the concentrations of a particular enzyme in a group of nerve cells, by means of a pseudo-colour programme. The panel at the right hand side of the picture shows the colour scale used. Areas of highest enzyme concentration are coded blue, and those of lowest concentration red.

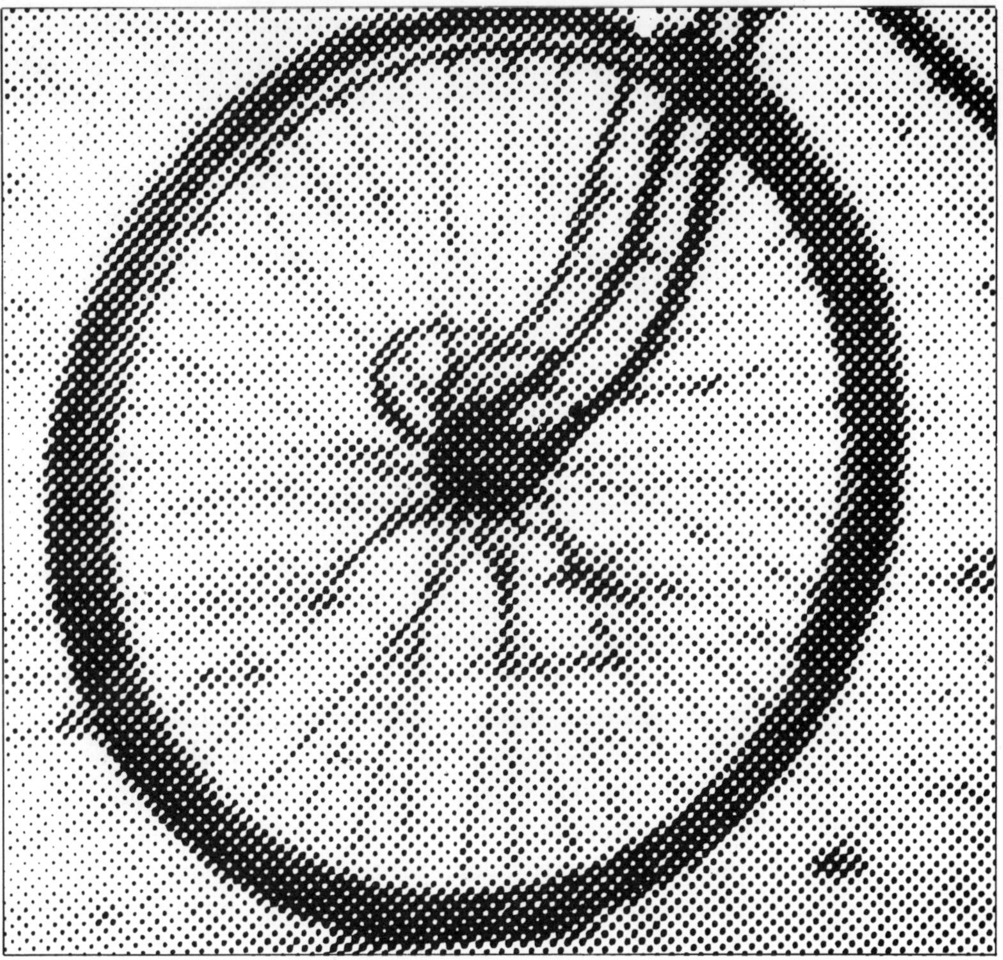

In the dark, our eyes see only with scattered groups of retinal cells. The image produced is rather like the dot pattern used in newspaper photographs, which is why things look blurred at night.

to light, the rods and cones are insensitive for a time. This is why a bright light shone into our eyes makes us temporarily unable to see clearly. When we look away from a bright object we sometimes still see its image, but now as a dark object on a pale background. The dark image corresponds to the area of inactivated retinal receptors.

The photopigment molecules present in the rods and cones of the retina all include vitamin A as part of their structure. An adequate dietary intake of this vitamin is therefore essential to vision. In particular, vitamin A deficiency reduces our capacity for seeing in dim light, causing night blindness.

Vitamin A is plentiful in egg yolk, dairy products and oily fish. It can also be made in the body from the pigment carotene, which is present in pumpkin, carrots and in the leaves of dark green vegetables. Both the vitamin and its precursor are quite stable to cooking and storage. In fact, a tin of carrots that was prepared for a British expedition to the Arctic in 1824 was opened in 1939 and found to have just as much carotene as fresh carrots. So, with a normal diet, deficiency of this vitamin is not a problem. But in some parts of the world, both fresh vegetables and animal products are a rarity. In these areas, an estimated quarter of a million children go blind every year because they do not have enough vitamin A.

Although all the photopigments found in the human eye are quite similar in chemical composition, the ones in the cones do vary in their sensitivities to light of different wavelengths. This provides us with the ability for colour vision. By contrast, the rods respond similarly to light of all colours. So in dim light, when vision depends entirely on the rods, we see in black and white rather than in colour.

Colour vision involves three separate types of cones, with photopigments that respond to red, green and blue light respectively. When we look at a coloureod object, the coded information that is sent to the brain contains a sprinkling of messages from each of these populations. The principle is just the same as three-colour printing in magazines, where many colours can be produced by mixing tiny dots of the primary pigments.

In most people who are colour blind, one of the three cone types is missing. Usually, the defect is in either the red- or the green-sensitive cones, so that these colours cannot be distinguished. This sort of colour blindness is usually seen in men, because the genetic information that determines development of the cones is carried on the male (Y) chromosome. Much more rarely, all the cone types are absent. These people rely entirely on the more light-sensitive rods for seeing, and so are easily dazzled by bright light, as well as being unable to discriminate colours.

While most of us can see equally well with either eye, binocular or stereoscopic vision is an important part of our ability to perceive three-dimensional space. If you hold your thumb at arm's length and look at it through your left and right eyes separately, you will appreciate that each eye sees any object

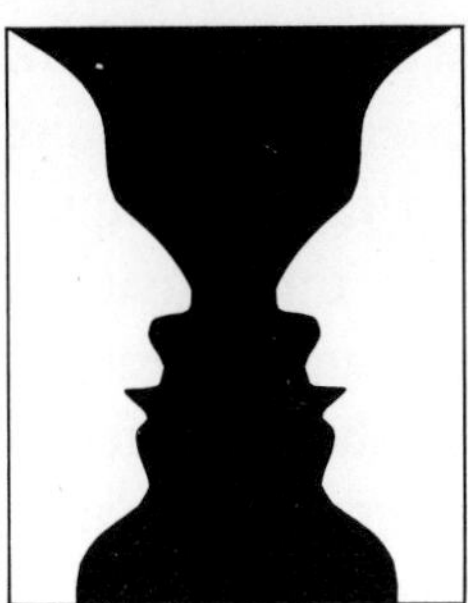

Is this a vase, or a conversation? Without more visual clues, it is not possible to decide.

from a different angle. This enables us to judge distance much more accurately. Usually, it is possible to pick up a small object like a paper clip or a thread from a desk top with a single movement. If you shut one eye, things may not look very different; but, now, accurate location of the object to be picked up may require you making some preliminary movements to work out just how far away it is.

Stereoscopic vision is also vital for recognising objects. When we can see a shape only in two dimensions, its identity is often ambiguous. Look, for instance, at the silhouette opposite. You can see a black urn, or, alternatively, two white faces. But, if you keep looking, these images keep interchanging. To see only one of the alternatives all the time, you would need some clue about what the picture looked like in three dimensions.

While our eyes detect the range of electromagnetic impulses that make up the spectrum of visible light, our ears detect the movement of individual gas molecules in the air. Some sounds, such as those generated by a tuning fork, are 'pure', that is, they consist of air moving at a constant frequency. However, most sounds that we hear are 'harmonic', consisting of mixtures of several or many pure sounds.

Sounds have three properties. Loudness depends on the number of air molecules in motion. The 'pitch', for instance, the notes C or A, describes the frequency of air movement. But notes of one pitch played on a piano are quite distinct from the same notes played on a violin. So we can also distinguish sounds by their 'timbre'.

The first stage in our detection of sound is the eardrum, a membrane that is stretched across the ear canal about one and a half centimetres in from the ear itself. Beyond the eardrum is an air-filled chamber known as the middle ear, and beyond that a second, inner chamber filled with fluid. This is also covered by a membrane. The actual detection of sounds occurs within the fluid of the inner ear.

The two membranes that make up the outer and inner walls of the middle ear chamber are connected by a series of three small bones that are hinged together rather like a piston. So movements of the eardrum caused by sound waves are transmitted to the fluid of the inner ear. Because the bones are hinged, and because the inner membrane is only about one-twentieth the diameter of the eardrum, the middle ear acts like a system of gears to amplify the eardrum vibrations. In fact, in a quiet environment, it is even possible to detect the tiny vibrations caused by blood flowing through the arteries around the ear.

If the middle ear chamber were sealed, then changes in atmospheric pressure would change its size and distort sound transmission. To avoid this, the chamber is connected to a narrow canal, the eustachian tube, which opens into the back of the throat. This tube is normally squashed shut by the tissues around the throat. But when one swallows, it is stretched open, and equalises the pressures in the middle ear and the atmosphere.

If our eustachian tubes become blocked, for instance by inflammation during a cold, then we may experience disruption to normal middle ear function as 'ringing in the ears' and distorted hearing. If atmospheric pressure changes suddenly, for example in an aeroplane, then swelling of the middle ear may cause pain. Repeated swallowing movements open the tube, and allow the pressures to equalise.

The inner, fluid-filled chamber of the ear contains rows of cells that have hairs upon their surfaces, sticking up into the fluid. Vibrations transmitted from the middle ear produce a pressure wave, which bends the hairs. This movement then opens up holes in the membranes of the cells, and charged ions diffuse across and produce electrical activity.

The hairs must be small and delicate, in order to be able to respond to small sounds. But this also means that they are easily damaged. Repeated exposure to very loud noises, such as amplified music, has been shown by electron microscopy to tear many of the hairs out of their cells, leaving large gaps in the range of sounds that can be heard. Unfortunately, unlike many types of cell, the hair cells never regrow. So the deafness that occurs is permanent.

As well as detecting sounds, the ear has a second function. Near the inner ear chamber, three other fluid-filled canals also exist, containing tufts of hairs. These canals are arranged so that they all run at right angles to each other. The hairs therefore separately measure fluid movement from side to side, up and down and from front to back of the head. The effect of gravity on this so-called vestibular system tells us how our bodies are oriented in relation to the ground. Movements of fluid that interfere with the gravitational signals can produce nausea, as occurs in motion sickness.

As well, the vestibular system helps us to balance while we are walking. Here, however, it is usually less important than some other ways of controlling balance. So long as they can see the surroundings, even people with an inactive vestibular apparatus are able to maintain balance adequately.

Our eyes and ears are used to help us know what is going on around us. They also help to protect our bodies from injury. But people who are blind or deaf learn to cope with the dangers of life very efficiently, provided that they have another, far more important, form of protection. This is the ability to feel pain.

Pain is the only way in which we can recognise damage to our bodies. Nerves in the skin that detect pain warn us to stop holding a hot saucepan before it burns us badly. The pain of a sprained ankle stops us using the leg, and allows healing to occur. Painful angina of the heart prevents us taking exercise, and so limits the amount of work that a sick heart has to do.

We are so used to automatically avoiding situations that cause pain that we easily forget just how important it is as a protective device. But some people lose the sense of pain because of degenerative nerve disease. And in others, the pain nerves do not develop before birth. These unfortunate individuals routinely suffer from horrific damage that they are unaware of, caused by broken limbs, deep burns and skin infections.

Pain sensation arises in very fine nerve endings, which respond electrically to pressure or local concentrations of chemicals. When inflammation occurs, this releases chemicals from the damaged cells, and these sensitise the pain nerve endings. So inflamed areas, such as pimples, are sensitive to even minor knocks that would not feel painful elsewhere on the skin.

Unlike the skin, internal organs such as the intestine can be cut or burnt without producing painful sensations. But the pain nerves in these organs do respond to stretching. So we feel unpleasant sensations when gas is trapped in the intestine, when a varicose vein is distended with blood, or when a bile stone becomes jammed in the bile duct.

The pain nerves in internal organs are also sensitive to the acid waste chemicals which build up when there is a local lack of oxygen. So blockage of the coronary blood supply to part of the heart muscle causes the severe pain of a heart attack. Oddly enough, this pain often feels as if it were occurring in the shoulder or arm, rather than in the heart. Physiologists think that this is because pain nerves from the heart and the shoulder both enter the nervous system through the same part of the spinal cord. Because we are used to recognising sensations coming from the body surface, but do not normally receive any sensations from the heart, our brains identify the pain stimulus as originating in the shoulder.

Headache is one sort of pain that can be caused by several different mechanisms. The most common sort of headache occurs because of concentration or emotional tension. Here, excessive contraction of the muscles that support the head blocks blood flow to these muscles, and build-up of acid wastes stimulates the pain nerve endings.

Migraine, by contrast, is caused by the stretching of pain nerves in the large blood vessels outside the brain, because they are distended by excessive blood flow. Yet a third type of headache is associated with hangovers. Here, the alcohol that has been drunk depletes water from the body and so causes the brain to shrink slightly. This stretches the structures that connect it to the skull, and pulls on pain nerve endings.

Household painkillers (analgesics) like aspirin prevent the formation of local chemicals which normally sensitise the pain nerve endings, so they reduce the number of electrical impulses that a painful stimulus produces. But they cannot prevent nerve activation entirely, so severe pain is not much affected. Narcotic analgesics like morphine, on the other hand, block the passage of pain messages within the brain. These substances therefore can prevent even severe pain.

During experiments on how narcotic analgesics prevent pain, scientists found that some brain cells contain natural substances which are very like morphine. These substances not only block pain pathways but also affect other brain activities including food appetite and blood pressure. So they may represent important physiological regulators in several parts of the brain.

SMELLING AND TASTING

Our ability to detect tastes and odours is likely to have evolved partly as a contribution to our survival; it may not be coincidental that most poisonous plants taste very bitter, and most toxic gases have a detectable smell. But, as well, taste and odour are an important part of our enjoyment of life.

We detect tastes through chemical stimulation of special receptors (taste buds) on the upper surface of the tongue. Four types of taste buds exist, the stimulation of which causes sensations of saltiness, bitterness, sourness and sweetness. These different receptor types are distributed differently: for example, sweet receptors are only near the tongue tip, so we cannot taste sugar if it is placed at the back of the mouth. You can easily work out for yourself the approximate distributions of the four taste bud populations by applying solutions of sugar, lemon juice, salt water and quinine to the tongue with a cotton bud. Make sure you rinse your mouth well every few minutes to stop the solutions getting mixed together.

Clearly, most of the flavours that we experience during eating are more than mixtures of these four basic taste sensations. Texture also alters the way we interpret food – warm icecream, for instance, is not particularly appealing. But even more important is the participation of our sense of smell. Everyone has experienced the fact that foods lose much of their expected taste if one has a cold and the nose is blocked.

The receptors that detect odours are located high inside the nose, almost between the eyes. When we breathe, most of the air travels through the lower part of the nose towards the lungs, so it may not reach the region around the receptors. Sniffing allows us to detect smells more easily, because it sucks air up into the top of the nose.

The mechanisms for detecting odour are much more

complicated than those for taste. As with the taste buds, different odour receptors are able to detect different smells, and so odours can be classified according to the type of receptor that they activate. But there is a good deal of controversy about how many receptor types exist. One popular theory is that there are just seven, described as floral (and typified by the smell of roses), ethereal (typified by ripe pears), pungent (like vinegar), putrid (like rotten eggs), minty, musky and camphor-like. By this theory, all the other characteristic smells that we know, such as aniseed, oranges or tar, result from activation of several of these 'primary' receptor types at once. Current thinking, however, favours the view that there may be additional groups of primary receptors that selectively recognise odours like sweat or urine. Yet more types may be discovered in the future; as the human nose can distinguish up to 4000 different smells, and interpretations of particular smells often vary from person to person, it is almost impossible to define the situation exactly.

Another puzzle about taste and odour detection is how the molecules involved are recognised. For instance, a solution of common salt (sodium chloride) is detected as salty, but the very similar molecule potassium chloride tastes bitter. Furthermore, it cannot be the sodium atom itself that is recognised as salty, because other sodium compounds, such as sodium bicarbonate (baking soda), are not salty tasting either. The most intriguing problem comes from observations in species other than man. Any stockman knows that cattle have an uncanny ability to sense when they are approaching water: this seems to be because they can smell it. And in rats and cats, the tongue has a special set of taste buds that respond selectively to water, rather than to one of the four standard tastes we can detect. Scientists have no idea of how a sensory receptor could recognise water in these ways.

Chapter Eleven

. . . and Looking Inwards

Our awareness of the world, and how we react to it, depends on the cerebral cortex, that wrinkled cap that gives the brain its typical appearance. The cerebral cortex is in fact a thin flat sheet of nerve cells, almost ten thousand million of them, and about the size of one page of a newspaper. But this is much bigger than the size of the head. So the sheet has been crumpled up, like a ball of paper, in order to fit it into the skull.

Particular areas of the cortex have a special ability to handle particular jobs. For instance, the part at the front of the brain is involved with producing the behaviour patterns that give us individual personalities. Just behind this is the area that co-ordinates muscle movements, and, behind this again, the area that receives information from the outside world. Some control areas are in surprising places. The visual cortex, which processes information from the eyes, is right at the back of the brain.

The two sides, or hemispheres, of the cortex also have rather different functions. For the brain to work normally, both sides need to be able to communicate with each other. Nobel prize-winner Roger Sperry discovered this in the 1950s when he studied a series of patients in whom the two sides had been separated surgically, in order to restrict the spread of uncontrollable epileptic seizures.

Although each eye is connected to both sides of the brain, the outer half of the retina sends messages only to its own hemisphere. Normally, this information can still travel to the opposite side, by pathways within the brain. But in Sperry's patients this connection was cut, so independent visual inputs could be sent to each of the hemispheres. Sperry seated his subjects in front of a tray containing an assortment of objects. The written name of a particular object was flashed to the outer half of one eye, and the subject was asked to pick up the correct item and name it.

The 'split brain' patients could identify and name an object so long as messages from the eye were received by the left side of the brain. But when only the right brain received the message, although they still picked up the correct object, they were unable to name it. These fascinating experiments show that both sides of the cortex can receive sensory information; and both sides can carry out motor tasks, like picking something up; but only the left side can communicate by means of speech.

The patients studied by Sperry had received no damage to the actual areas of cortex needed for speech. But, in some people, strokes may damage the nerve cells that interpret language patterns and transform thoughts into words. These people are in a doubly tragic situation. As well as being unable to communicate, their inability to speak or write means that they are usually regarded as mentally subnormal.

The processes described above, of recognising objects and speaking, rely on information stored in our memory. This has drawn attention to the similarity between the brain and a computer. However, there are in fact some very important

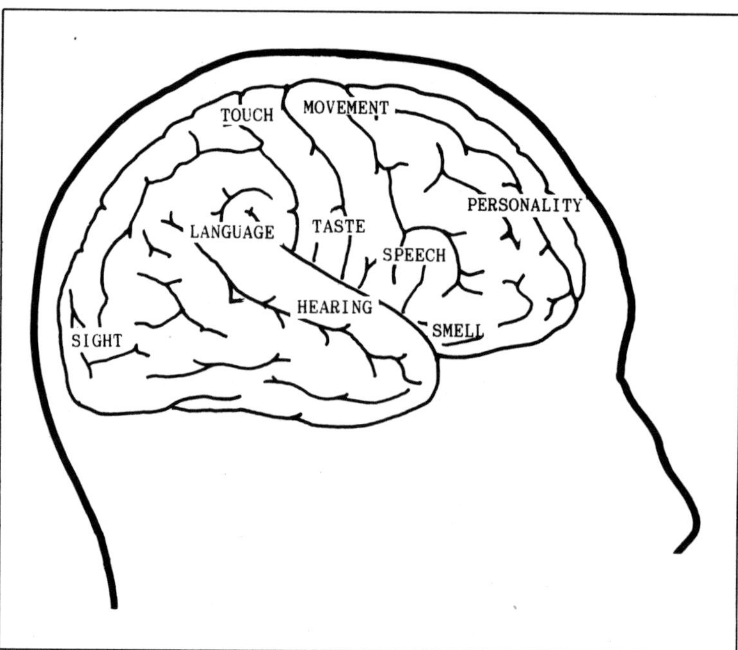

Different parts of the cerebral cortex have distinct functional roles.

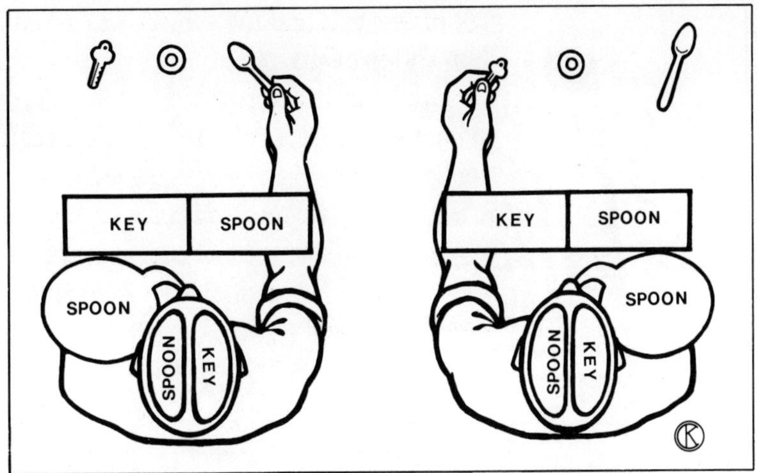

Spoken language seems to be a property only of the left hand side of the cerebral cortex. Here, in the classical experiment performed by Sperry, a split-brain subject has the written word 'key' directed to the right side of his brain, and the word 'spoon' directed to the left side (note that under the conditions of the experiment, information entering each eye travels only to the opposite side of the brain). He is then asked to select the named object from the table in front of him, using each hand in turn. When the hand controlled by the right brain (the left hand) is used, the object selected is the one shown to that side, but the subject names the object shown to the left brain.

differences between the ways in which these two systems handle information.

First, the amount of information that can be stored in a computer depends only on the size of its memory. But we remember something complicated better when it is presented bit by bit than all at once. A computer retains information in the exact form it is entered. But we remember generalities far better than factual details. Finally, computer storage requires a piece of information to be entered only once. But our memories are more likely to last when they are reinforced by repeated exposure.

This reinforcement process seems to move the memory from a 'short-term' to a 'long-term' store. For acquired skills, like learning to read and write, the memory is virtually permanent once the transfer has occurred. In fact, there may be a third sort of store especially for these complex memory patterns.

Short-term memory almost certainly involves local electrical circuits, so anything that disturbs electrical activity in the brain, like a blow on the head, may destroy recent memories. Long-term memory does not depend on electrical impulses. It probably involves structural changes in the nerve cells, in the same way as foreign antigens induce immunological memory by stimulating specific receptor sites on white blood cells (see Chapter 3).

Much of our ability to cope with everyday life relies on being able to remember our experiences. People who have lost the part of the brain necessary for memory can only live from moment to moment, and every experience is lost again almost immediately.

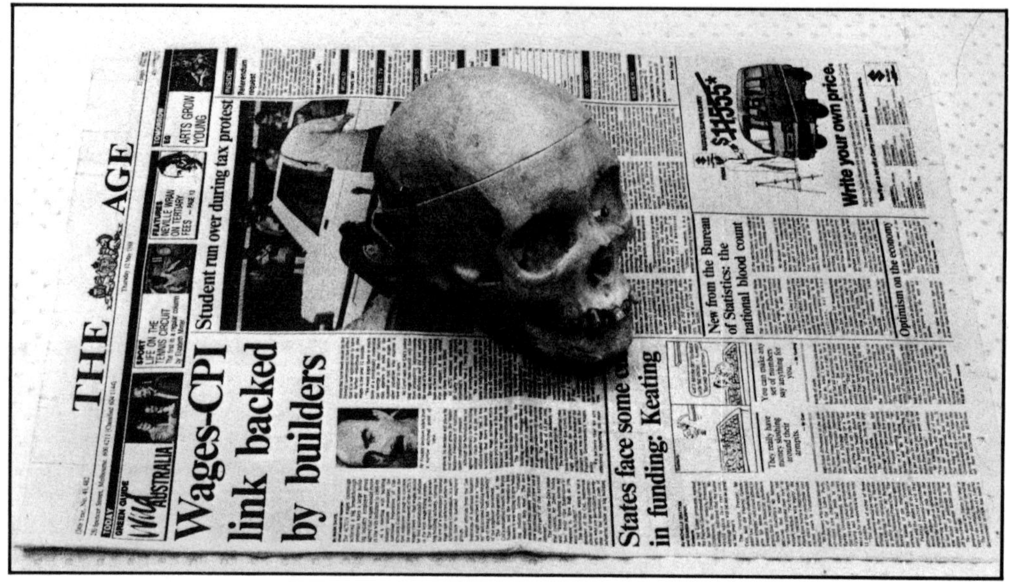

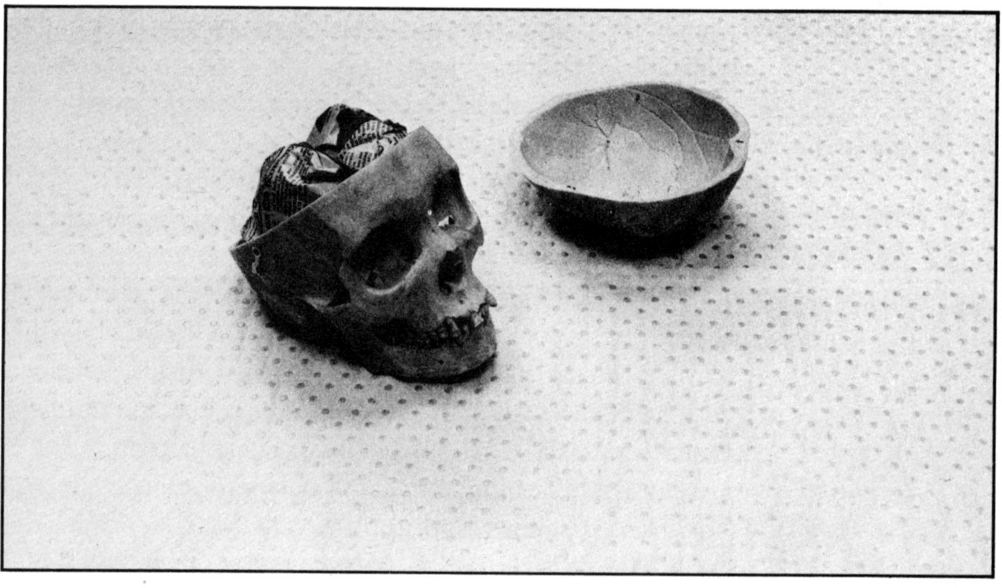

If it were spread out flat, the cerebral cortex would be about the size of a sheet of newspaper.

But even a perfect capacity for memory is useful only when we can appreciate what is going on around us; in other words, when we are conscious.

Electrical activity in the cells of the cerebral cortex can be measured by recording the voltage difference between points on the scalp overlying particular areas of the brain. The recording obtained is the electro-encephalogram, or EEG. This activity decreases with anaesthesia or coma, and during sleep. So we can say that consciousness is at least partly located in the cerebral cortex. It is less certain what controls the transition between wakefulness and sleep, and what the significance of such different states of consciousness actually is.

If a person is totally deprived of sleep for several days, the psychological and physical effects are dramatic. However, the number of hours slept each day can be greatly reduced without having any adverse effect. And Siamese twins with the same blood circulation show independent sleep patterns. So set periods of sleep are apparently not necessary for removal of accumulated waste products from the body, or for cell repair. One alternative theory is that sleep is needed for proper memory processing: perhaps for removal of data that are no longer needed, or for transfer of memories into permanent stores.

Some periods of sleep are deep, and EEG activity is much reduced. But other periods are associated with EEG patterns that are very like those occurring when we are awake. At these times, the eyes flicker back and forth, so these periods are known as 'rapid eye movement', or REM, sleep.

People woken from REM sleep usually report having had a dream, while most of those woken from deep sleep have not been dreaming. If a person is selectively deprived of REM sleep by being woken every time eye movements are seen, the percentage of sleeping time spent in REM sleep increases. We seem, therefore, to need REM sleep more than deep sleep. At one time, this was thought to indicate that dreaming is an essential biological function. However, people who have been selectively deprived of REM sleep for months do not appear to change psychologically, so the importance of dreams is still a mystery.

Although consciousness is localised in the cerebral cortex, it originates in nerve cells that lie far deeper, in the base of the brain. These cells act as a switch, which turns the cortical consciousness on during waking hours and off while we are asleep.

English physiologist Colin Blakemore pointed out in his 1976 Reith Lectures that this arrangement may have important philosophical and ethical implications. Brain death is usually defined as loss of nerve cell activity in the primitive centres deep in the brain that control functions such as breathing. At this time it is assumed that death has also occurred in the rest of the brain. But death of the primitive centres may itself switch off consciousness. So a brain could, in theory, retain all its cortical functions, without the means to express them.

Throughout this discussion I have been using 'consciousness' very simplistically, as a distinction from unconsciousness. Thus, it implies an awareness of the environment, and the capacity to respond to it. But by this definition, even simple animals like jellyfish are conscious. It is obvious that for higher animals, and especially for human beings, the terms of reference are considerably more complex.

Science can explain the basis of awareness, if by this is meant the ability to sense physical and chemical changes. Neuroscientists may soon understand how we sense that some changes are dangerous and some are innocuous. But what is the biological basis for awareness of the differences between a painting by Van Gogh and one by Cezanne? Equally, a response to the environment could mean escaping from danger: even primitive organisms do this, and work on the nerve pathways in creatures such as leeches will soon provide the circuits involved. But human responses to many environmental stimuli are much more complex. How does the scientist begin to understand the mechanisms that are involved in, for example, the appreciation of beauty?

The concept of personality is more complex again. In previous chapters, we have seen that many human behaviour patterns are designed to maintain the body's internal environment. For instance, we drink when we feel thirsty, to compensate for water losses in the urine; we put on clothes when we feel cold, as part of the processes that maintain body temperature. But a lot of the things we do cannot be explained away as reflex responses. Which shoes we decide to wear, which foods we order in a restaurant make up a very important part of our lives and contribute to our individual personalities, but have no survival value.

Some of these responses probably occur because we learn to act in certain ways, to achieve a pleasant result. Experiments with animals have shown that the hypothalamus of the brain contains nerve cells that act as a 'reward centre'. When miniature electrodes are implanted under anaesthesia into this part of a rat's hypothalamus, and the rat is taught to use a switch to stimulate the reward cells, it spends most of the day doing this.

It is not known whether the more complex human pleasures, like enjoyment of a piece of music, involve the same nerve pathways. Interestingly, however, we do know that these sorts of responses can be stored permanently within the brain. When areas of the cortex just behind the forehead are stimulated electrically in conscious patients, they vividly recall past experiences. This storage seems to be quite distinct to normal memory, because there is only recall of emotionally oriented experiences, like listening to music.

The external expression of personality depends entirely on the frontal area of the brain. Our awareness of this stems from a remarkable accident that occurred during the building of a railroad in Vermont in the autumn of 1848. While the foreman of the blasting team, Phineas Gage, was tamping down a charge, it exploded, driving the iron tamping rod up through the front of his head. To everyone's surprise, Gage survived. But his personality had completely changed: formerly an easy-going friendly man, he was now surly and argumentative.

This sort of personality change is now known to be a common result of frontal brain damage. Such patients are also unable to master simple learned tasks, like sorting out different shaped objects. Their disability is not because they cannot remember. Instead, there is loss of some filter that normally limits the rate at which messages are received by the brain, with the result that it is swamped by the amount of information arriving. There is some evidence that very much the same sort of problem also exists in autistic children.

Although most of what we know about how personality is expressed has come from observations of the results of trauma to the brain, the mechanisms that determine personality can become disturbed without any signs of physical damage. The most common of these personality disorders, or psychoses, are schizophrenia and depression. Most of the medicines that are useful in treating these diseases modify the activity of one particular chemical messenger, a substance called dopamine, and for this reason, some physiologists have suggested that all psychoses are caused by too much or too little dopamine in the brain.

In fact, as the same medicines are useful in different illnesses, which are distinguished by quite different behavioural disturbances, it seems unlikely that a single cause can be evoked. The role of dopamine is probably in the expression of personality, rather than in its basic character. Nevertheless, the fact that a particular chemical messenger has been implicated at all is one of the very few pieces of biochemical evidence that we have about cortical function.

So we have come back full-circle to the conclusion reached at the end of Chapter 1 of this book: that, despite the enormous advances made over the last one hundred years in particular, science is still a long way from grasping the complexities of human brain function.

This is partly because of the intricacy of the system involved. New techniques for identifying and studying particular nerve populations, such as immunological cell labelling and computerised brain scanning, are currently helping to resolve some of these difficulties. Another problem is how to attack questions like the basis of personality, using experimental techniques. In contrast to other areas of physiology, animal experimentation is of only limited use here, because of the uniquely human nature of the characteristic being studied.

Some philosophers propose a third limitation to these investigations, by suggesting that, by definition, a mind can never completely understand itself. One thing, however, is clear. No matter how much we find out, it can only enhance our feeling of wonder for the reality that is inside ourselves.

PERCEPTIONS OF REALITY

A disruption of the pathways that link different areas of the brain can lead to bizarre changes in the relationship between perception and interpretation. Michael Gazzaniga at Cornell University has recently been studying split-brain patients similar to those which were discussed in the main text of this chapter. One patient was shown a series of pictures, which included a chicken's foot and a snow scene, and was asked to match them with a second series, which included a chicken and a shovel. When his left brain was shown the chicken's foot, he selected the chicken picture. When his right brain was shown the snow scene, he selected the shovel. But when asked to explain the choices, he said 'Oh, that's simple. The chicken's foot goes with the chicken, and you need the shovel to clean out the chicken shed'. Although the left side of his brain responsible for spoken communication did not know why the shovel had really been selected (because the relevant visual clue only travelled to the right brain), it immediately made up a logical explanation.

Another patient with a quite different problem, but one still related to a breakdown of the links between perception and understanding, was described by Oliver Sacks *in his fascinating book 'The Man Who Mistook His Wife for a Hat'. This man could describe what he saw, but was not able to interpret its meaning. Shown a glove, for example, he identified it as a container with 'a continuous surface infolded on itself (and) five outpouchings', and thought that it might be a purse for five different sized coins. The suggestion that it was an item of clothing was met with disbelief. He could remember the plot details of books, but not the visual descriptions in them, nor the emotional implications. So, while his memory as such was unimpaired, he was unable to use it to make useful judgements about reality.*

Given these graphic demonstrations of the ways in which our brains can mislead us, it is tempting to speculate on the possibility that less severe damage of the types described above may explain some personality traits. Are some habitual liars in fact unable to distinguish truth? Is a 'lack of imagination' a sign of a minor disruption of the pathways completely destroyed in Dr Sacks' patient?

Sources of Illustrations

COLOUR ILLUSTRATIONS

FOLLOWING PAGE

16 University of Melbourne Medical History Museum. Courtesy Prof. H. Attwood.
Black-throated Robin, watercolour & pencil, J. Cotton, 1843–1848. Courtesy La Trobe Collection, State Library of Victoria (MS 9817, plate 44A).
Black Thursday, February 6th, 1851, oil, W. Strutt, 1864. Courtesy La Trobe Collection, State Library of Victoria (LT 990).
Richmond Volunteers' Regiment, albumen silver photograph, Batchelor & O'Neil, 1861. Courtesy La Trobe Collection, State Library of Victoria (H 22044).
Wannon Falls, chromolithograph, N. Chevalier, 1865. Courtesy La Trobe Collection, State Library of Victoria (LTAEF 19).

48 Barium radiograph. Courtesy Dr N. A. Davis.
Eagle's View of the Mountains: Head of the Mitta Mitta, oil, E. von Guerard, 1879. Courtesy La Trobe Collection, State Library of Victoria (LT 211).
Courtesy University of Melbourne Department of Physiology. Photograph by Reinier Mann.
Commercial Travellers' Association menu. Courtesy La Trobe Collection, State Library of Victoria (H 35715).

96 *Natives Discovering the Body of William John Wills, the Explorer, at Cooper's Creek, June 1861*, oil, E. M. Scott, 1862/4. Courtesy La Trobe Collection, State Library of Victoria (LT 944).
Constitution Hill at Sunset, From Near Mrs Ranson's Public House, oil, J. Glover, 1840. Courtesy La Trobe Collection, State Library of Victoria (LT 1039).
Red Fury, John Vickery, c. 1970. Courtesy Charles Nodrum Gallery and Mrs J. Vickery.
S.S. Toroa, watercolour, A. V. Gregory, 1908. Courtesy La Trobe Collection, State Library of Victoria (LT 652).
Invalid Digger, watercolour, S. T. Gill, c. 1854. Courtesy La Trobe Collection, State Library of Victoria.

TOP: *St Francis*, wax painting, Cinello, c. 1980.
MIDDLE: Model courtesy Dr David Story. Photograph by Reinier Mann.
BOTTOM: Courtesy Dr Chandan Gurusinghe and Mr David Ashburner. Photograph by Reinier Mann.

BLACK AND WHITE ILLUSTRATIONS

PAGE

3 Imaginary portrait, from Robinson, V., *Pathfinders in Medicine*, Medical Life Press, New York, 1929.
5 Engraving by W. Faithorne, after the bust by C. Jansen in the Royal College of Physicians. From Harvey, W., *On Generation*, London, 1653.
6 Woodcut from Harvey, W., *Movement of the Heart and Blood*, Frankfurt, 1628.
7 Photograph courtesy Wild Leitz (Australia).
8 Courtesy the Department of Physiology, University of Melbourne.
10 Drawing after the statue by Guillaume on the steps of the College of France. From Bernard, C. *Arthur de Bretagne*, G. Barral, Paris, 1887.
16 Transmission electron micrograph. Courtesy Meredith Ferguson.
20 Courtesy the Department of Physiology, University of Melbourne.
21 Drawing by Cam Knuckey.
22 Reproduced from *From Neuron to Brain*. Courtesy Sinauer Associates Inc. and Prof. J. Nicholls.
25 Courtesy the Department of Physiology, University of Melbourne.
26 Scanning electron micrograph. Courtesy Dr Daine Alcorn.
28 Scanning electron micrograph. Courtesy Geraldine Kelly.
32 Data from *Oxford Textbook of Medicine*, 1983.
34 Commercial model of circulation marketed by Baird Tatlock, London, c. 1910.
35 Photograph by Reinier Mann.
36 Material courtesy the Department of Physiology, University of Melbourne, and the University of Melbourne Medical History Museum. Photograph Reinier Mann.
37 Scanning electron micrograph, reproduced from Fujiwara, T., *American Journal of Anatomy*, 170, 39–54, 1984. Courtesy Allan R. Liss Inc. and Dr Fujiwara.
39 Photograph courtesy the *Age* newspaper.
45 Photograph by Reinier Mann.
46 Courtesy the Department of Physiology, University of Melbourne.
47 Scanning electron micrograph. Courtesy Dr Daine Alcorn.
52 Scanning electron micrograph. Courtesy Dr Daine Alcorn.

55 Kathleen Curnow, member Australian Underwater Hockey Team. Courtesy University of Melbourne Underwater Club. Photograph by Nathan Richter.
58 *Browne's & Smythe's Mining Company, Smythesdale,* c. 1861, Solomon & Bardwell. Courtesy La Trobe Collection, State Library of Victoria (H 20366).
59 Scanning electron micrograph. Courtesy Miss Anastasia Gabriel.
68 Etching from German anatomical text, c. 1700.
70 Drawing by Cam Knuckey.
72 Courtesy the Department of Physiology, University of Melbourne.
80 Photograph courtesy the *Age* newspaper.
87 Emigration poster, c. 1834. Courtesy La Trobe Collection, State Library of Victoria (H 31022).
89 Reproduced from *From Neuron to Brain.* Courtesy Sinauer Assoc. Inc. and Prof. J. Nicholls.
90 Hilltop castle, Arraiolos, Portugal.
92 *General Tom Thumb in Western Australia*, albumen silver photograph. Courtesy La Trobe Collection, State Library of Victoria (Copyright collection).
107 Drawing by Cam Knuckey.
108 Skull courtesy Department of Physiology, University of Melbourne. Photograph by Reinier Mann.

Index

Aboriginals 82–3
'acquired' immune deficiency syndrome (AIDS) 30
action potential 16–17
ageing 91–3
alcohol 60, 81
alcoholism 62
alveoli, lung 45
Alzheimer's disease 86
anaemia 25–6, 31–2
angina 40–1, 42, 101
animals, research on 4, 56, 93, 110–11, 112
antibodies 24, 29, 41
aortic aneurysm 34
appetite 63
arteries 33–8
aspirin 102
asthma 46
ATP 20–1
autistic children 111

balance, sense of 101
bile 61
binocular, or stereoscopic, vision 98–9
blood cells 24
blood clotting 24, 27–9, 61
blood pressure 9, 33–40, 42, 69
blood-brain barrier 41
body temperature 77–85
bone marrow 31
bones 73
brain, functions of 105–13
brain death 109–10
breath-holding 51
breathing 44–56
breathing underwater 54–6

calcium 24, 73
cancer 30–1, 86
capillaries 33, 41
carbon dioxide 25, 48, 50–3, 74
cerebral cortex 105–13
chemical messengers (see neurotransmitters)
colon 58–9
colour vision 95–8
colour-blindness 98
common cold 30
complement 30
computer, differences of brain from 106–7
congenital defects 86
Conn's disease 69
consciousness 108–10
constipation 59
convulsions 74
cot death 52–3
curare 9

deafness 100
decompression 55–6
dehydration 60
depression 111
development (see growth)
diabetes 63, 67
diarrhoea 60
digestive tract 57–62
diphtheria 29
diving 54–6
dizziness 37–8
dopamine 111–12
'dowager's hump' 74
dreams 109
drowning 45

eardrum 99
ears 99–101
electro-encephalogram (EEG) 108–9

emphysema 47
energy expenditure 62
erythrocytes (see red blood cells)
eustachian tube 100
exercise 53, 62, 69
eye 95–9

fainting 38, 47
fatness 61–4
fevers 84
fibre 59
flushing 40, 79, 83
food additives 75

gene cloning 11–12
genes 31
genetic defects 32
glaucoma 96
glucose 24, 61, 63, 67
growth 86–91
growth rates 91, 94

haemoglobin 25, 48, 61
haemostasis 27
hangovers 102
head injuries 69, 111
headache 42, 102
heart attacks 29, 72, 102
height, increase with growth 89
hepatatis 60
high altitudes 49
high blood pressure (hypertension) 35–6, 54, 72
histamine 41
hormones 24, 35, 41, 63, 69, 73, 77
hypertension (see high blood pressure)
hyperthermia 84
hyperventilation 51
hypothalamus 110–11
hypothermia 85

imagination 113
immunity 24, 29–31
infection 24, 29, 30, 41
insect bites 41
insulin 63
interferon 30–1
intestine 57–60
ions, definition of 15
iron, need for 26

jaundice 61

kidney 67–74

learning 12
leucocytes (see white blood cells)
liver 60–3
lungs 44–8, 50–5
lymphocytes 30

malnutrition 60, 91
memory 12, 106–7
metabolism 1, 62, 79
metabolites 40
middle ear chamber 99–100
migraine 102
morphine 102
motion sickness 101
multiple sclerosis 17
muscle contraction 19–22
muscle movements 105
muscle weakness 17
myelin 17

nerves 15–19, 86–8
neurotransmitters 17–19, 88, 111
night blindness 98
nitrogen 55
noradrenaline 35
nutrition 57–8, 64, 89

obesity 54, 63, 66
oedema 61
osteoporosis 73
ovulation 77
oxygen 25, 48

pain 40, 101
painkillers 102
pancreas 63
parathyroid glands 73
Parkinsonism 86
perception 112
peristalsis 59
personalities 12, 105, 110, 113
pH 51, 74
pituitary 69, 91
platelets 24, 27
pneumothorax 44
poliomyelitis 29
posture 81

potassium 15, 24
pregnancy 48
premature babies 45, 50, 56
psychoses 111
puberty 94
pupil of eye 96

'rapid eye movement', or REM, sleep 109
red blood cells 25, 48
retardation of growth 91
retina 96
'ringing in the ears' 100
rickets 74
rigor mortis 22

saliva 58
salt (see also sodium) 36, 67, 71, 79
schizophrenia 111
SCUBA diving 54–6
shivering 79, 83
Siamese twins 109
skin temperature 80
sleep 52, 54, 109
smoking 46
snoring 52, 54
snorkel divers 51
sodium (see also salt) 15, 24, 75–6
space craft 50
speech 106
'split brain' patients 106, 112–13
stinging nettles 41
stomach 57
stroke 12, 29, 42, 72, 106
sweating 79
synapses 17

temperature control 77–85
tetanus 29
thalassaemia 25, 31
thalidomide 88
thirst 67, 71
thrombi 28–9
thyroid gland 91
trachea, or windpipe 46

urine 67, 69, 71, 73, 74

vegetarians 26
veins 38
viruses 30
vision 95–9
viamins 61, 64–5
  folic acid 26
  vitamin A 96, 97
  vitamin B_{12} 26
  vitamin D 73

water balance 58, 79
weight ranges, ideal 65–6
weight reduction 63, 65
white blood cells 29–31, 41
wisdom teeth 90

yawning 45, 51